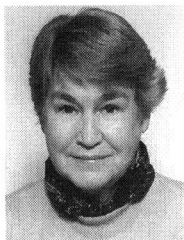

MARGARETE
as an interna
seminars on co
ship. She is tl
People and Organizations (2004), *Time for Transformation* (2008, with Hans Stolp) and *What Happens When We Die?* (2017). For more information visit her website: margaretevandenbrink.nl

MORE PRECIOUS
THAN LIGHT

How Dialogue can Transform
Relationships and Build Community

MARGARETE VAN DEN BRINK

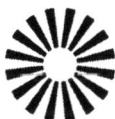

TEMPLE LODGE

Translated by Tony Langham and Plym Peters

Temple Lodge Publishing Ltd.
Hillside House, The Square
Forest Row, RH18 5ES

www.templelodge.com

Published by Temple Lodge Publishing 2021

Previously published in English by Hawthorn Press 1996
Originally published in Dutch under the title *Verkwikkender dan licht*
by Uitgeverij Vrij Geesteslevern, Zeist, Netherlands 1994

A CIP catalogue record for this book is available from the British
Library

ISBN 978 1 912230 78 5

Cover by Morgan Creative featuring an image by Hans Geissberger
    used by permission of Raffael-Verlag, Switzerland
Typeset by Floris Books
Printed and bound by 4Edge Ltd., Essex

Contents

Self knowledge and change

Paths to Christ

'Where do you come from?'

'From the subterranean passages where gold is found', said the snake.

'What is more precious than gold?' asked the king.

'The Light', answered the snake.

'What is more refreshing than light?' asked the king.

'Conversation', said the snake. *

* From the *Fairy Tale of the Green Snake and the Beautiful Lily* by J. W von Goethe, translated by Thomas Carlyle, in Paul and Joan Allen, *The Time is at Hand,* Anthroposophic Press, New York, 1996

Foreword

This conversation is taken from *The Tale of the Green Snake and the Beautiful Lily*, by Goethe. In lively images and conversations, this tale describes the path of initiation leading to the mystical wedding, the unification of the human self with its higher, spiritual being. In order to achieve this, there has to be a transformation in everyday man, or as Goethe said: 'One has to surrender one's existence in order to exist.' The Gospels talk about rebirth in the same sense.

In this initiation process, conversation plays a central role, as Goethe indicated. Why is this, and why does it act in a way that is more invigorating than light? This is related to the mystery of the word. In certain circumstances, the words which people speak to each other contain a force which works in an invigorating and life-enhancing way. Although Goethe does not give this force a name, it is clear that he was talking about the highest creative principle, the creative word, which is also referred to in the *Gospel According to St. John*, and which created everything that exists.

Once, the divine world influenced humanity from the outside, filling human thoughts, feelings and acts, as well as words, with divine power. In the world of the *Old Testament* or of the *Vedas*, the word still had an inner force. It had a suggestive and magical effect. When man spoke, it was as though an angel, a higher spiritual being, was talking along with him. These words had healing powers, but could also be damning.

In the course of human evolution, words lost more and more of their spiritual content and power. The word, and consequently human consciousness, lost its divine content. This was a necessary process, for without this loss, we could never have become independent and free. We would always have remained under the influence of divine and spiritual forces. In order to gain inner freedom, words had to lose their spiritual effect, and had to become increasingly hollow and empty.

It is as though the deepest point of this process has been reached in our own time, and a change of direction is taking place. More and more people are looking for a way of connecting with the divine. This new connection can be made because the God who is known as the creative word, the Logos, made this possible at the beginning of our era. He took the path of initiation, the path of inner transformation, and followed it to its ultimate conclusion. He incarnated in a human body and passed through a process of death and resurrection. In this way he cleared a new inner path towards the divine world for every human being on earth.

Christ, the creative word, is the divine force which in the past worked from the outside. However, since Golgotha, he lives in man himself. He is waiting in our soul until we develop him in us. If we seek him there and give him life within us, our words will gradually once again be filled with the divine creative force and become active in the contact between people, no longer in a magical, restricted way as in the past, but consciously aimed at liberating the other.

Regaining the lost power of the word was – and is – the aim of every true path of initiation. Goethe showed us the way in the images of his fairy tale. For him too, the means to this end is dialogue, in interaction with another person, through words. He explained that if we develop the potential in our soul and our love for the world, we will thus gain ever greater insights and arrive at truth. Not only is more and more of our higher self born in this way, but at the same time we also resurrect Christ, the creative word, in our self, and give him life. The more we do this, the more our words will lose their emptiness. They will become meaningful, and filled with the power of the Logos, they will have a healing and liberating effect on others.

The path of development which Goethe revealed in the image of his fairy tale was described by Rudolf Steiner in the concepts of the spiritual science of anthroposophy. He described the path of the human being to his higher spiritual being, and thus to higher levels of consciousness and existence, in many different ways.

This book was written on the basis of anthroposophical insights. It indicates the path towards the spirit and towards the lost power of the word, of Christ, in contemporary images and words. In addition, I have endeavoured to formulate the insights based on anthroposophy and to relate these to real life in such a way that it is possible to identify with them, and to test them with one's own experiences.

I would like to thank the Non Nobis Foundation for giving me the financial opportunity to write this work, as well as Frans van Bussel from the Uitgeverij Vrij Geestesleven for his co-operation during the process of completing the book, and all the people with whom I had essential conversations and which so contributed to the development of this work.

Margreet van den Brink

.

New Times

Life is changing

All around us we can see that life is changing. All sorts of customs and views, values and norms, which had told us for generations how we should think, feel and act are losing their force and are disappearing. This change is most obvious in the field of traditional belief. The influence which the church had for centuries on what people do and how they think has virtually disappeared. Everywhere, in families and at work, in the street and in politics, life has a different colour from the past. At the same time that this loss of traditions is taking place, we also see decay, decadence and increasing violence all around us.

However, far-reaching changes can be seen not only in society, but also in ourselves and in our relationships. Everyone has their own experiences of periods of inner crisis, a sense of alienation from their partner, an inner void which cannot be filled.

And yet, all these experiences of feeling uprooted, and all these changes, also have a positive side and significance. For in addition to uncertainty, they also give rise to an inner need to discover new answers to the age-old questions: Who am I? Where do I come from? Where am I going? What is the meaning of life?

We search around to find what is at the back of it all. Some are more concerned with the background of their own lives; others more with that of 'life' in general. We find that something new is stirring in our inner being, something which leads us to become active ourselves. We find that we are no longer willing to unquestioningly accept what experts or authorities pronounce or prescribe. We want to understand things for ourselves, find out what is good and what is not, and decide for ourselves what we will do. We discover a need for working on ourselves in order to become more complete. For we feel that it is only when we become more complete that we are able to relate better to our partners, our children and our fellow human beings.

It is clear that far-reaching changes are taking place in people at the moment. Some people have said that it seems as though a spirit of inner renewal is working in and between people, and that its presence is tangible.[1] So what is happening?

The cosmos is changing

Rudolf Steiner, who was able to perceive the spiritual forces behind external events, describes the evolution of mankind and the earth as a development towards ever higher levels of consciousness and existence. During this evolution periods of far-reaching change and renewal occur. Our own age is one of these stages of renewal, which will result in human development reaching a higher plane.

What happens during this stage of change and renewal? We gain an insight into this only when we take into account the fact that specific spiritual forces are at work behind the development of mankind and the earth, consciously directing its evolution. In the Christian tradition these spiritual forces behind the evolution of the cosmos are known as God the Father, God the Son, and God the Holy Spirit. They operate independently, but nevertheless form a unity: as the Three-In-One or Divine Trinity of creative form, life and consciousness, they permeate and carry the universe and everything that exists.[2]

The Father is the indication of the supportive principle in the cosmos, the 'basic foundation' of existence. It is possible to imagine that once divine forces flowed from the Father into the universe, ultimately creating the material substance of the cosmos, gaining a solid form in nature and in man.

The Son is the true creator of the world, the fundamental source of everything that becomes and develops in the cosmos. If the Father is he *from* whose forces all existence has come forth, the Son is the divine force *through* which everything was created.[3] *The Gospel According to St. John* explains this. St. John calls God the Son, 'the Word': 'In the beginning was the Word, and the Word was with God, and the Word was God. The same was in the beginning with God. All things were made by him, and without him, was not anything made that was made.' [4]

However, the existence and substance of all the phenomena we see around us not only come from the Father and gain life and development through the Son, but also contain 'Spirit'. The effect of the third creative principle, the Holy Spirit, is expressed in the meaningful order, the wisdom and harmony of that which we find in nature as a whole and in every single creature.

The first stage of evolution – the offshoots of which we experience in our own time – was characterized particularly by the Father. The world of the Father manifested itself not only in external creation, but also in the soul and in the consciousness of humanity. In the course of time, this consciousness evolved from an archaic universal consciousness through a magical and a mystical stage towards a groupbound 'We-experience'. In none of these stages did man experience himself or others as separate individuals. [5] Everyone still felt at one with the world around him, or later, with the group to which she or he belonged. This is clear from all the ancient texts and traditions which tell us about the development of mankind, like, for example, *The Old Testament*. This describes how God led his people by choosing certain figures to govern the lives of the nation, tribe or family group in accordance with the given norms and values. These leaders determined what people should think and experience, and how they should act. Moses's Ten Commandments are an example of this. There was not yet any question of any inner personal freedom.

Although we nowadays still frequently come across vestiges of behaviour determined by leaders, authorities, or the group, we see that in the last century more and more people try to free themselves from these old religious and social traditions, and follow their own individual paths. It is clear that something that lives deep down in the souls of human beings is ready to develop. This means at the same time, that the work of the Father is coming to an end. Higher divine beings, the angels, who, directed by the Father, have led human and earthly evolution since ancient times, are now withdrawing.[6] The result of this is that we as people are no longer naturally bound to each other, and that all the ancient forms of society, which are based on man as a groupbeing, are falling apart. We face each other now as independent individuals and have to discover new ways to find each other.

These changes take place not only on the level of the soul and in social life, but there is also the withdrawal of the old spiritual forces from nature, including the human body. The entire physical material world is in a slow, but irreversible process of decay. The fact that the creation of God the Father is a mortal, finite world, is also clear from the fact that nothing new is being added to this world. On the contrary, it is constantly losing parts. No new rocks have formed, nor new plants, animals or human types. Existing rocks are eroding into dust, and species of plants and animals are constantly disappearing. Also the sun is in a slow process of extinction. However, this gradual death of the material world has a deep significance. The spiritual forces from the plane of the Father, which carried evolution up to a certain point, are now withdrawing to make room for different divine forces which will give creation a new, spiritual, substance, and this will lead mankind in a new way. This does not mean that the divine Father himself will cease to exist, but that his relationship to creation has changed.

From the time that the divine beings from the plane of the Father began to withdraw from evolution, the forces of evil, the counterforces, spread throughout all creation. In addition to their operation in the souls of man, they also work in material nature and thus in the human body. Because of the ever-growing influence of the counterforces in creation, the earth and mankind are in danger not only of decaying at an ever-increasing rate, but also of being irreversibly cut off from the divine world. In order to deflect this threat and enable the progress of human development, the divine Son, Christ, came down to earth and united himself with creation.

This is the awesome fact hidden behind the mysterious events which took place between Good Friday and Pentecost, two thousand years ago. In these events, which are described in anthroposophy as 'the mystery of Golgotha', Christ went through the process of death and resurrection, and was born *in* the earth, *in* mankind, and *in* every single human being. This sacrifice of the divine Son means that he from then on permeates the physical world with his new creative forces from within, and in this way saves it from destruction, including the human body. At Ascension, Christ then penetrated the etheric sphere, the sphere of life forces, which permeates everything that lives, finally to descend into the soul and the I of every single human being on earth during the event of Pentecost.

The event of Pentecost took place when the disciples were gathered together in Jerusalem, following Christ's Ascension. Then the wind sweeps through the house and the Holy Spirit, springing from Christ himself appears and in the form of fiery tongues enters each of them individually. At that moment, the disciples and with them every single person on earth becomes the bearer of a new seed: the spirit of Christ, the active, creative, spiritual aspect of Christ, the Christ-impulse.[7] With Christ the Word, the Logos force, but also divine love itself entered creation and the souls and I's of human beings. In this way the Son's scope of operation, which had been limited during the first stage of creation to the external world of nature, now expanded into the soul and the spirit living in the soul.

When the Spirit which Christ had sent descended, the disciples experienced a tremendous process of inner awakening that started in the head and ended in their limbs. In the first place, they were now able to understand the truths which Christ had been teaching them for three years through their own spiritual activity, their own active thinking. After their capacity to think actively for themselves was awakened, their speech was liberated. They now not only could find and think truth for themselves, but could also express and broadcast it. From there, the forces of Christ's love descended even further: into their hearts and into their limbs.[8] This meant that they could now speak to other people in their own language, cure their diseases, free them from evil influences, and awaken them in their deepest inner being. At the same time, they felt that as the disciples of Christ who experience truth and love in themselves, they were bound together as brothers in a new independent way. The descending Spirit released forces in them as individuals, as well as new social forces. The Spirit of truth and love enabled them as apostles to go out into the world, preach about the workings of Christ, to cure the sick and to awaken and release in people the new supportive forces of the spirit.

In our own time the spirit of Christ becomes increasingly active in us in a way similar to that which took place in the disciples two thousand years ago. We can already experience this process in ourselves and in our contacts with other people. It is part of the new impulses that nowadays stir in our souls, though we do not yet recognise these as such.

Christ's aim in coming to the earth has two aspects: on the one hand, he wants to renew the mortal, physical substance of the world of the Father, through his Spirit and on the other hand, he wants to awaken every single human being inwardly and connect her or him with her or his deepest spirit being. In our time we experience this working of the Christ in our soul as the need to know the truth about ourselves, and about the people and things around us, but also in impulses to develop feelings of warmth and love. When we respond to these impulses and become inwardly active ourselves, a process of transformation will take place in our soul in which our higher spirit self, filled with the power of Christ, comes forward ever more clearly. The central issue in this development is, as we can see, the necessity to become inwardly active in our thinking, our feeling and in our will.

Then the words spoken by Christ in the *Book of Revelations* will be fulfilled: 'Behold, I make all things new. [9] The transforming power of Christ will then gradually receive the opportunity to create a new heaven and a new earth, as well as a new mankind. And so the development of mankind and the earth will not be destroyed through the process of decay but will continue in a new way on ever-higher levels of existence.

To summarize: on the basis of the above, we can distinguish three aspects in the working of the divine Spirit, the Divine Trinity. In the first place, there is the divine Spirit who formed the physical-material basis of all creation. He can be recognised in the divine wisdom and harmony that permeates all that is visible.

Secondly, we find the divine Spirit in what Rudolf Steiner calls 'the Christ-impulse': the Spirit of Christ, God the Son, who since Golgotha lives in the earth, in humanity as a whole and in the soul and I of every single human being. This Christ-impulse, the active working of the Christ-spirit, not only arouses the higher being in the soul when the individual becomes inwardly active her- or himself, but through that process also renews creation in decay.

Thirdly, the divine Spirit lives and works in us in a twofold way as God the Holy Spirit. He lives in our soul as our own higher spirit self and works in us from the outside via our thinking, our capacity to penetrate the reality of the world around us and in us and to understand the truth that lies hidden there. The next chapter will deal especially with the mystery that is connected with the thinking.

The working of the Spirit in us

We saw how, since Golgotha, and in particular since the first Pentecost, humankind has been connected with the divine Spirit in a new way. This confronts us with the question: how does the spirit work in each of us individually today? In order to gain an accurate picture of this, we should start with an understanding of how people are formed and how this process works.

As human beings, we have a body, a soul and a spirit. The spirit is our true being, that which goes from one incarnation to the next. In every new life it builds up a new soul and a new body, and thus also a different personality. At the present stage of our development this true spiritual being cannot yet live entirely in our body and in our personality. This is possible only when the latter have been transformed into suitable vehicles or instruments. In order to achieve this, we keep returning to earth and during all our different lives we transform a little more of our physical nature and personality. That is why, in general, at the beginning of every new life there is a slightly more suitable vehicle for the spirit than at the start of the previous life. This means that our true being is able to live and work on earth a little more effectively after every new birth.

In Anthroposophy this higher spiritual being is referred to as the spiritual self or spirit self, the higher self or Self, or simply as the individuality. The spirit self is part of the sphere of the Holy Spirit, and therefore also has the same properties.[10] These properties are an infinite consciousness, strength, wisdom, harmony and goodness. In the distant future we will be able to express all these qualities through our human form. Our spiritual being will then be able to live on earth in all its glory in a suitable physical body and personality.

In our own time this spirit self wishes to develop further in us, as our most essential individual aspect. All the changes and turbulences which we experience in ourselves and in society are related to this.

How should we perceive ourselves in this development of the spirit self? It is possible to understand this development properly only when we realise what I mentioned before, that the spirit self works in us in two different ways. It works from the outside and from the inside, in the same way as the divine Spirit of which it is part. The external part hovers largely still over us, living in a general, unindividualized form in the spiritual world. It is that part of us that we have not yet become, but that we are in the process of becoming. It expresses itself in our faculty to think and understand.

The part of our spirit self which lives within us is completely different. Steiner called this the inner or the higher human being. This spirit self was formed in its essence in our physical nature at the very beginning of creation. Since then, it leads a dormant existence in the deep unconscious layers of our being, until it awakens.[11] To some extent this awakening has already taken place. In the incarnations behind us, parts of this inner human being developed gradually. This process also continues in our present incarnation. Therefore Rudolf Steiner made a distinction between those parts of the soul in which the spirit self is already active, and those parts in which it is still 'asleep'.[12] Where the spirit self has already been partly awakened in us, we are able to express an essential and individual part of ourselves. In this case, we have already become ourselves to a greater extent. This can be experienced in abilities which we reveal, in the clarity of our consciousness, in the wisdom, inner strength and stability, that we have acquired and in goodness that we have developed, and so on.

This inner self develops when we have experiences and learn from them. These experiences we have during the day we take with us into sleep. There they are transformed, in our absence so to speak, into skills and abilities and into qualities which gradually become manifest in us in the course of time. Rudolf Steiner often gives the process of learning to write as an example of this transformation. As a child, we learn to write with a great deal of difficulty, trying again and again. However, later on we do not remember anything of all our efforts and experiences during this learning process. They have been assimilated into the ability to write, i.e., the ability to express thoughts on paper. This ability then expresses an aspect of our own essential spirit self.

The transformation of our experiences results not only in physical skills, but also in an enlargement of our consciousness, or in inner strength. This happens as follows.

When we ask ourselves a question and then think about it, we will, sooner or later, come up with an answer or an insight. This answer comes from the content of the consciousness of the spirit self which works inside us, and is then caught up by our thoughts.[13] This is how it becomes conscious to us. It is then scrutinized by our feelings to see whether it is true or not. If it is, it is assimilated into our I, and from that moment becomes part of us. This makes the I or the personality a little wiser. In other words, there then comes to life a little more of the consciousness and the strength of our inner spirit self in our soul and in our personality.

These examples show us that there is a direct link between the spirit self which works from the outside, and the spirit self developing within us. When we become spiritually active, i.e., when we start to think about things and in this way gain understanding, discover the essence of things and find truth, the spiritual being slumbering within us is awoken by this activity. The deeper the insight, the greater the awakening. The same thing happens when we try to change and improve qualities of our soul through a process of self knowledge.

The transformation of the soul and the awakening of the higher being which takes place when we consciously deal with our experiences in this way happens through the activity of the spirit of Christ which lives within us. He is the great transformer. In one of his lectures, Rudolf Steiner said: 'Everything which man can take from his personality as a fruit for his individuality is given him because he has a link with the Christ.'[14] This means that there is also a close link between our inner self and the Christ impulse living within us. I will return to this later.

The need which people feel nowadays to become aware of things, to find truth themselves, and to change and develop themselves, indicates that it is this inner spiritual being who wants to come through in our time. This is what is knocking at the door of our inner selves asking for attention and integration. This is what inspires us to ask questions and look for answers, seeking the truth about our lives and life in general. After all, it is only through the inner activity which we engage in that the spiritual human being within us can be awakened.

Personal and social development

In this day and age, the desire for the spirit self, the spirit person in us, to break through, is expressed in two different ways: in the first place, in the need to develop the individual personality as strongly as possible, developing the spiritual powers within it; and secondly, in the need to be there for people other than oneself, and to help them in their development. In this respect I make a distinction between the individual impulse and the social impulse.

The individual impulse means that we are primarily geared towards ourselves and our own development. This is a necessary endeavour because we have to become an independent personality, and transform ourselves into a suitable instrument for the spirit. When we do this in an honest way, i.e., working on ourselves on the basis of sincere self-knowledge, something strange happens. For when the power of the spirit is released in our personal development, it also arouses the other, the social orientation. The development of the spirit self awakens within us the profound need to truly understand other people and to have concern for their needs.

This is because the spirit self developing in our inner being is not only part of the Holy Spirit but is also permeated by the spirit of Christ.[15] These both have an individualizing effect as well as the effect of connecting people together through the power of consciousness, the power of love based on knowledge. The experiences of the disciples at Pentecost serve as an example of this. When the Holy Spirit descended upon them they each individually became a personal bearer of the Christ-impulse on the one hand, while on the other hand, this power from Christ connected them to each other and to other people in a new way. The same also applies to us ordinary people. When we truly understand something about another person, this always evokes a desire within us – as a result of the effect of the Christ-impulse – to help that person in some way, and support that person in his or her development. Essentially the social impulse *is* the Christ impulse working between people.[16]

The individual impulse, which is aimed at the individual's development, endeavours to help the person to attain increasing inner strength and richness. This is right, because it is the task we have been given to perform. In this sense we *should be* 'selfish'.[17] However, there is always a danger that we could start to follow an unrealistic and one-sided path in this individual development. For example, it is tempting to develop only our strengths because this makes us feel good, or because this enables us to influence others. The dishonest angle resides in the fact that we then choose not to look at our weaker aspects, or that we do not want to become aware of the extent to which we owe our stronger aspects to other people. This results in a distorted development. We become increasingly imprisoned in ourselves, living only for our own development, our own needs, desires and ideas. In the end it is possible to lose all meaningful contact with the world around us.

On the other hand, we should not make the mistake of seeing every impulse to take an interest in other people, or helping them, as the effect of the social impulse. In fact, this sort of 'social' attitude often conceals a desire for recognition by others, a need to hold on to a certain self-image, or a way of experiencing oneself. The same causes are at the basis of the tendency to seek common ground and associations in conversations with others, rather than seeing the other person as he or she truly is. In this case there is no true encounter with that other person. Ultimately this apparently social behaviour in contacts with other people leads to problems which are every bit as great as a one-sided individual attitude. It is only when we develop in a way that allows the spirit self to be released within us that we can transcend the one-sided nature and needs of our I. When the spirit self develops we also gradually develop the ability to truly understand things and people, and thus discover truth in an objective sense: a truth which transcends the subjective 'personal' truth which still separates us so distinctly from other people nowadays.

The mystery of evil

Up to now I have referred only incidentally to an important factor in the history of mankind and in the life of every individual: to what is traditionally known as 'evil'. In our own time, when a new movement towards spiritual insight, truth and morality is becoming apparent, it seems as though tendencies such as indifference, callousness and violence are also becoming increasingly evident. What are the forces behind this and where do they come from?

We saw that during the earlier stages of human evolution, humanity was still to a great extent led by the spiritual world, but that this direction from the world of the Father has gradually receded. This withdrawal of the forces of the Father made way for the forces of evil. As a result, people on earth were less and less able to experience their divine origin. In the course of their incarnations they were drawn down by these forces deeper and deeper into the world of the physical body and earthly material things. The passions, and therefore selfish elements, were aroused, and consciousness narrowed. Mankind started to wander and people allowed themselves to be led by egoism and illusion. However, getting lost in this way and being caught in the grip of evil is inextricably linked to man's path to freedom.

In fact, getting lost and encountering the forces of evil means that we wake up to ourselves. By constantly being confronted with the question of what is right and what is wrong, and by discovering the effects of good and evil for ourselves, we actually find ourselves as well as learning to understand these two forces. In this way we become aware of what we really want, and thus of our true being. It is only thus that we are free to choose the forces which we wish to use in the world. The mystery of evil is that because of the resistance that it brings about, the goodness that is consciously wanted can be expressed up to its highest form.

Spiritual forces or spiritual beings are concealed behind the evil tendencies. Originally, these beings came from the highest ranks of the divine hierarchies. However, in the very distant past they turned away from the divine world and followed their own path. They did this with the intention of facilitating the development of mankind towards independence. Therefore their act formed part of the divine plan of creation.[18] By taking on this task, these higher beings made an inconceivably great sacrifice. They gave up not only the world of light, harmony and bliss, but also chose a life abandoned by God. The further they became distanced from the divine world, the more their consciousness darkened. Their deep, unfulfilled longing for the divine world changed direction and turned in on themselves. They became trapped in themselves and in their own endeavours.[19] A revulsion and hatred for everything that was divine, unselfish, true and good developed in them. Since that time they have been intent on gaining power over the spiritual forces which reside in man and nature, and to use these for their own purposes and for the expansion of their own power. These beings, which are the opposite pole to the effects of the beings of light are known in Anthroposophy as the counter-forces or the counter-powers.

On the basis of his studies of spiritual science, Rudolf Steiner distinguished different sorts of counter-forces. The best known are Lucifer and Ahriman, known in *The Bible* as Diabolos and Satan, which each lead particular groups of spiritual beings.

The force known as Lucifer aims to free mankind from all earthly things, to imprison him in a sort of spiritual world of his own making. He does this by arousing the need in the human being to constantly feel and experience her- or himself, on the level of the soul as well as spiritually. He encourages us to have or to know more, to be higher, better or more important than other people, and to experience oneself in this elevated state. Lucifer leads us to things which are higher than ourselves, including high moral and spiritual ideals. However, the problem is that he does this in such a way that we separate ourselves from everything which is still impotent, undeveloped, 'earthly' or bad in ourselves, which we then ignore. As a result, qualities such as arrogance, pride, vanity, and so on, develop. Lucifer creates an inner schism: there is the tendency to identify with the higher aspects and to ignore or deny the lower.

In addition to Lucifer, Ahriman is also a leading counter-force in our time. Lucifer raises man up above his own level; Ahriman casts him down. He wants us to separate ourselves from the spiritual world and to identify completely with earthly material reality and with our lower nature. He achieves this by means of narrowing the capacity for thought and consciousness. Thus he deceives us into thinking that the ordinary earthly personality with all its shortcomings and selfish aims is man's true nature. He confronts us again and again with our weak and rather base sides to show us that we are worthless human beings. Ahriman does not acknowledge anything such as the spirit, truth, morality and inner development. The spiritual world does not exist; it is an illusion. Man is no more than a higher animal. His spirit is no more than a biological computer, and therefore death is the end of everything. The only 'truth' is what can be quantitatively demonstrated, and all else is 'subjective'. In fact, Ahriman preaches the meaninglessness of life. In this way, he not only evokes a sense of impotence and depression in human beings, but also an existential feeling of fear. Deep-rooted fear results in hatred, and this is the next aspect evoked by Ahriman: mockery, cynicism and hatred for everything which has value in life, everything that is true and good.

At an even deeper level, hatred becomes a force of destruction. This brings us to the essence of the third elementary counter-force, the Asuras or Asurian forces. The Asuras wish to destroy everything that exists, on the level of the physical as well as on the level of the soul and the spirit, and want to use the spiritual forces that are thus released for themselves. These high beings from the region of the counter-forces endeavour to arouse the basest instincts in men, the urge to abuse other people physically or spiritually, to hurt them or even destroy them, and to derive pleasure from doing this. Like the Ahrimanic forces, the Asurian forces gain access to people particularly in situations where consciousness is lowered or extinguished, and the instincts and passions are whipped up.[20] In such situations, people are lifted out of themselves, and thus these forces are able to descend into them and affect the world through them. The Asurian forces are still at the beginning of their development in the souls of mankind.[21] Their influence is gradually increasing, and will reach its high point in a later age.

Obviously the counter-forces affect events in the world and the course of history through people. For example, the effect of Lucifer can be recognised in all sorts of nationalist movements with special group interests born from a feeling of superiority to others, or in societies governed by a dictator where the elevated Luciferian position of the leader is usually accompanied by an Ahriman-like suppression of individual freedom. In fact, because of his tremendous influence on science and technology, Ahriman is the great inspirator of modern culture.

The counter-forces have access to us because, as the world of the Father withdraws, this leaves 'spaces' in us which are not yet filled with substance of the spirit self.[22] However, there are parts of our physical nature, and of our soul, which they cannot penetrate. These are the parts of our I or personality in which the rough substance of the soul has already been transformed into the spiritual substance of the higher self, through Christ. The counter-forces cannot affect this inviolable, imperishable substance of our true self.

In our own time at the end of the twentieth century, the struggle between the forces of light and darkness is reaching

a sort of peak. More than ever before, we are active participants in this struggle. Human development has progressed
so far that the definitive step to the spirit and spiritual
transformation must be taken in every field of life. Therefore
the forces of evil are now mustering their troops to prevent
this. However, behind the shadows cast by them, a powerful
light is shining.

The working of Christ in our time

Christ, God the Son, once lived on earth, as a man of flesh
and blood. He lived through the events of Golgotha and so
conquered the death of matter. In this process he carried the
basic form of the physical body – the force field which holds
the substance of the body together – through death and
resurrection and in this way saved the physical body for all
mankind from decay.[23] During the short time between
Easter and Ascension when he lived on earth in a visible
form, he lived in this so-called resurrected body. In this
spiritual body he was able to appear everywhere, to make
himself known to people and to speak with them.

This came to an end with his Ascension. From the time
that he 'ascended to heaven', his body could no longer be
perceived even by his followers. However, Rudolf Steiner
pointed out that Christ's ascension did not mean that he left
mankind and the earth to depart to a distant place in the
cosmos. In fact, this would have conflicted with his promise
that he would remain with people until the end of time.[24]
Christ continued to be linked to the world and to the people
into which he had descended and continued to work in
there. With his Ascension he expanded this influence and
entered the wider spiritual regions which permeate and
surround the earthly world. His activities in these regions
meant that he was not visible for a long time.

However, in our own time his connection with us as
'ordinary people' has progressed so far, partly as a result of
our own development, that he is gradually appearing again
and is experienced by and is even visible to increasing
numbers of people. Now, he does not appear in the form of
a man of flesh and blood – his appearance in a human

physical body could only take place once – but in a spiritual, etheric body.[25] He manifests himself in this etheric body because, just as he was active in the earthly world in the past, he is now active in the etheric world. The etheric world is the sphere which permeates and surrounds mankind, nature and the earth with life forces. This etheric world reaches up to the level of the clouds. It is from this world of the etheric life forces that Christ will gradually become perceptible and even visible. Thus the prophecy will be fulfilled that he will come back on the clouds.[26]

This new manifestation will go so far that he will appear to people personally and will be experienced and even become visible to groups of people. Rudolf Steiner recounts how this miraculous event, the encounter with Christ himself, will happen to increasing numbers of people from the second half of the twentieth century onward. This is because people will become increasingly clairvoyant in a natural way. This will not only enable them to perceive the living bodies of plants, animals and people, but also that of Christ. In a number of his lectures, Steiner indicated how this will happen, and what form it will take.[27]

Man will be able to see etheric bodies, and will also be able to see the etheric body of Christ, which means that he will gain access to a world in which Christ will appear for his newly awakened abilities.

It will no longer be necessary to prove the existence of Christ with the help of all sorts of documents, because there will be eye witnesses of the presence of the living Christ, people who experience him in his etheric body. This experience will teach them that this is the being who went through the mystery of Golgotha, two thousand years ago; that it is Christ. Just as St. Paul was inspired with certainty at Damascus at that time: This is Christ – there will be people whose etheric experience will assure them of the fact that Christ is truly alive.

This is the greatest secret of our era: the secret of the return of Christ.' [28]

In another lecture Steiner says: 'These people will receive proof of one of the greatest statements in the *New Testament*, and they will be completely overcome. For in their souls the following words will be uttered: "I will be with you every day until the end of the world," which means, correctly translated: "Until the end of time on earth." This statement tells us that Christianity is not merely something which was written down in books once upon a time, and was learned during a particular era, that Christianity is not merely something summed up in certain dogmas nowadays, but that it is alive, comprising the experience and perception of revelations which will continue to develop more and more powerfully. Today, we are only at the very beginning of active Christianity, and anyone who has truly joined Christ knows that this Christianity will produce more and more new revelations. He knows that Christianity does not move backwards, but that Christianity is actively developing forwards; Christianity is not dead – it is alive.'[29]

In a lecture in 1911, Steiner indicated that in a few decades time, people would be in a certain place and experience something, and would then realize that someone would suddenly be there or would come to help them, and that Christ would be present in this person. Anyone who experiences this will think at first that it is an ordinary person of flesh and blood, but he will become aware that it is a spiritual being because it will suddenly disappear again. [30]

Christ will not appear only where people have to be shown something or when they want to know something. He will also be experienced when people are in difficulties or are suffering. The following experience will come to a person when she or he feels oppressed: '...when he sits in his room in silent sorrow and in despair, the door will open: the etheric Christ will appear and will speak words of consolation to him. Christ will become a living source of consolation to human beings!'[31]

'(...) The figure of Jesus Christ will approach him from the hidden depths of existence, and become the powerful force

in which he shall live, supporting and guiding him as a
brother ...' 32

In our own time, more and more people tell of such
encounters with Christ which have had a profound effect on
their lives. Some have described this experience in a very
individual way, such as in this poem by Hans Stolp: 33

The long-awaited one

It was evening and quiet. The day slid
Away from me. Then I heard a voice
Which asked: 'What do you see?'
I looked, and saw
The blinding light of heaven
Which came closer. Wide as a cloak,
The joy with which it clothed us from afar.
In that light a face.
Do you know that face? asked the voice.

I looked again. And knew. The long-awaited
Brother who is known to us by many names.
See, he comes, said the Voice.
Never before did I see a face
So full of love and goodness. Never before,
Had I been so happy. Then the light went out.
My room came back to me. But in me
The joy remained, and the reflection of the light.

Christ appears not only to individuals, but also to groups of
people who have gathered together for one reason or
another. They may be people who are in trouble and do not
know how to go on, or who are seeking insights into certain
problems or questions concerning life together. There too,
Christ may appear and participate in the discussions, visibly
or invisibly, giving insights and advice. This too is happening
in our own time. The following event shows how his
participation can be experienced.

A group of people who are greatly concerned with the social needs of our time had come together to study certain questions. After a difficult morning, in which many human obstacles had to be overcome, there was a discussion in the afternoon about the question of how the social impulse of Anthroposophy could be defined. The french windows into the garden were open; it was a warm autumn day with no wind. Suddenly a gentle breeze blew in, and then disappeared again. Shortly afterwards, something happened which could be seen as an inspirational event. One of the participants said something which appeared to have come from the depths of his inner self. Another was moved by this and contributed a new viewpoint, which also appeared to come from the depths of her soul. Then a third person said something which took these viewpoints even further. This process went on with others. Then it stopped. However, the process went on again when someone raised a new question on the subject. Again, fundamental insights on the subject came forward spontaneously one by one. The whole event gave the impression as if a source of inspiration was moving from one person to another, became active there, and then 'jumped' to another. Not only did the various answers fit together perfectly, giving a step-by-step insight into the question, but the answers also proved to be living experience. Someone said: 'Now I know by my own experience the spiritual meaning of the term "community"'. However, there was more to it than this. The event continued to affect the souls of the participants in a very special way. Afterwards, most of them described that they had experienced a deep sense of harmony and inner peace, the acceptance of their own and other people's mistakes and imperfections, and a feeling of connection with something much deeper in themselves. At the same time, this sense of unity miraculously also gave a sense of a deep connection with all the other people present.

These are some of the examples of the events which we can expect in our own time, now that the world of the spirit and of Christ has come so close that we can experience it.

Meeting and conversing

The individual path and the
social path to the spirit

The aim of the process of transformation which must take place in each of us is to find within ourselves the direction for our lives. Up to now, this has always been outside us. Nowadays we must strive to find the strength and support which have disappeared in the outside world within ourselves. This means that we must try to unite with the forces of the spirit self awakening within us. We must take the path inwards into our own soul and arouse the spiritual being concealed there. This is not an easy path to follow. It is strewn with pain, difficulties and obstacles. On this path to the inner self, we encounter all sorts of old certainties, patterns of thought and ways of acting which hinder the development of our spirit self. We will have to recognize these obstacles and resolve them. Anyone facing this task will be aware that it means going through a period of chaos where there is little or no support, without knowing where you will end up. This is a frightening experience, and may lead to a desire to leave everything as it is. However, without the death of this 'former person', the new spirit self within cannot be born.

By the 'former person', I mean the ordinary, everyday personality. This personality is our inner baggage, our inner equipment, which partly helps and stimulates us and partly acts as an obstacle. For example, the complexes and set patterns of response which we have developed in relation to the people around us and to the events in our lives are an obstacle. These one-sided and distorted qualities and patterns of behaviour to a large extent influence our thoughts, our feelings and our behaviour. This means that our personality is full of things which are not yet our true self. If the spiritual aspect wishes to develop within us, we must become conscious of these obstacles and transform them in such a way that our personality, as well as our thoughts, feelings and will, become a suitable instrument for the spirit.

Rudolf Steiner referred to this process of becoming aware in his book *Occult Science*.[34] He wrote that we must raise up the spiritual aspect from the depths of our soul by means of our own activities, so that we become conscious of it, and he continued: 'With the perception of the I – with self-reflection – starts the inner activity of the I.' Thus, by reflecting on ourself, i.e., on the soul content of our I, the power of the spirit self can start to work within this I.

Rudolf Steiner indicated that there are two aspects of the path to the spirit: an individual and a social aspect. By this, he meant that the inner human being can partly be aroused by ourselves, while the other part can only be aroused if the conditions for this are created in the contacts and interactions with another person.

The *individual path* is the task to reflect again and again on what is happening in ourself, so that we can get to know ourselves. At the same time, we should endeavour to develop the forces of our soul, our behaviour and our feelings and thoughts in such a way that they become an instrument for the spirit to work through. The individual path requires study and spiritual deepening. This is the nourishment for the spiritual being within us, and provides us with the insights we need in order to understand everything related to these new spiritual aspects.

Steiner describes this individual path in his book, *How to Know Higher Worlds*,[35] amongst other works. In this book he gives all sorts of ideas, exercises and meditations which result in the correct transformation of our thoughts, feelings and acts, allowing the spiritual forces to enter. These exercises and meditations gradually establish an increasingly strong connection between the ordinary self and the 'higher human being', as Steiner refers to the spirit self in this book.

At a certain point, this connection can lead to an enlightening experience. Then the person concerned suddenly becomes aware of the spiritual world living in nature, or all at once experiences some of the strength or the existence of his own higher being. We can follow this path ourselves without the help of others. To do so, we do not withdraw from life, but conceive the relationships with other people and the situation of our lives as a task, an exercise, for our own spiritual development.

As a result of this process of inner deepening and constant exercise and inner activity, the individual path transforms the soul forces into suitable instruments for the spirit. In this way the best conditions are created for following the second path, which may be referred to as the *social path*. This second path is aimed at awakening the spirit in the soul by means of encounters and conversations with other people. Rudolf Steiner described this path more clearly at a later stage in his life, and referred to it in a number of places. The aim of this path is to help each other to know our own self, and the soul of the other, and in this way awaken the living spirit, the spirit self in the soul.

Our soul or personality consists of an infinite number and diversity of 'contents': feelings, thoughts, needs, impulses, experiences, ideals, desires and so on. These are related in the first place to the events we have experienced since birth, and the encounters and relationships which we have had with countless people throughout our lives. Secondly, they are related to the situation in which we find ourselves at the moment. Thirdly, in the form of needs, desires, impulses and ideals, they are also related with what still has to develop within us. We refer to the total content bound up with our past, present and future, as the 'I'. This is the content of our own I-personality, our ordinary ego.

In the midst of all these experiences, needs, impulses, ideals and so on, our spirit self lies hidden and dormant. If this spiritual being is to be awakened and to become active, we must 'unpeel' it as it were, from all these experiences of the soul, and liberate it, so that it can be experienced. This happens when we come to understand the essence of all these stirrings in the soul: when we gain an insight into the true meaning of a particular situation or experience, and when we understand what we really want or wish to express or reach.

However, it is not possible to go through this process on our own. To do so, we need each other. This does not mean that we cannot gain an insight into our experiences ourselves, or cannot gain an awareness of what we want – we certainly can. However, the problem is mainly that we are not in touch with a large part of the experiences, needs and impulses living in the soul. In the natural way of things, we have contact only with a very limited part of ourselves. This conscious layer is rather thin. Most experiences gradually sink deeper and deeper into the unconscious layers of the soul, and are ultimately stored in the etheric body, or even in the physical body. This disappearance of experiences, for example, by repression, can go so far that we forget them entirely and no longer have any access to them at all. On the other hand, there are all sorts of impulses, desires and ideals living in our superconsciousness which are related to the development of what we have to become in the future, and these are also difficult to reach.

We are dependent on the concern of another person to help us to open up the inaccessible subconscious or super-conscious parts of our soul. This concern is the key. When another person is interested in what is happening to us, listens to us and asks questions, creating the space for us to express ourselves, we not only become familiar with a larger part of our soul, but we also come closer to our own spirit self. This produces new inner strength.

It is easy to observe how this concern works when we ourselves ask someone else about his or her experiences, desires and ideals, and explore these. In the first instance, there is often a sense of surprise that this is happening. Clearly people are not used to it. They may try to establish how seriously the questions are meant and how much space there is for an answer. This sort of explanation and assessment takes place because everyone knows that after one or two questions, most people start to talk about themselves and are no longer interested in the other person. However, when the other person continues to express an interest, this leads to some inner movement. We see a change in the facial expression, often the face gains colour, the eyes become livelier and sometimes shining, and it is evident that a lot is happening in the soul. These phenomena occur in any person we talk to in this way, whether it is a shop assistant at the greengrocer's, a conductor on a train, or a professional colleague in a dialogue.

When the soul starts to stir, the spirit self is activated and becomes more deeply incarnated, as it were, in the body. Often the hands and feet get warm, and there is a sense of inner enthusiasm and delight. At the same time, this is accompanied by a clarity in the soul. By expressing what is happening to them, people become aware of the dormant aspects in their soul and are in closer contact with themselves.

This incarnating and awakening effect is reinforced when we not only respond to the other person's experiences and impulses in an empathizing and interested way, but also gradually start to formulate insights on the basis of these. These insights may express the true nature of what is felt, or reflect the essence, so that the other person thinks: 'Yes, that's how it was, that's what I experienced, that's what the experience was about', or 'That's what I really want, that's what I'm aiming at.'

When this insight is achieved in the right way, i.e., when the insights arise from the situation itself, and are not imposed upon it intellectually, the other person feels that he comes closer to himself. He makes contact with a deeper part of himself, and this produces a sense of liberation and strength. This reveals that a little more of the spirit self has been awakened in the I. The inner being is awakened by consciously focusing on the content of the soul in this way - interacting with another person – and by permeating and enlightening it with knowledge and insight. In his book, *Die Mystik (Mysticism)*,[36] Steiner wrote: 'Thus a perception of oneself is at the same time the awakening of the Self.' After such meetings people sense that inwardly something has changed. After talking together in this way, someone once said to me: 'More of me is present now.' This describes exactly what is happening. People who have experienced this awakening of their individual being feel that they have become more harmonious, stronger and freer. They are revitalized by the influx of spiritual forces into the soul. In this way more of their mortal being is transformed into the immortal substance of the Spirit.

Light in the soul

What actually happens to us when we hold conversations and relate to each other in this way? In order to understand this, it is necessary to know a little more how the soul works and how the spirit self develops in this.

Our soul consists of three separate layers of consciousness which developed one after the other during the course of human evolution. The oldest part of the soul, the part which is still strongly connected to the life processes of the physical body, is known in Anthroposophy as the sentient soul, or sometimes, the soul of experience. Our deep subjective needs, emotions, impulses of the will, and so on, live in this part of the soul. These form the subjective basis, as it were, for our perceptions of the outside world. Through the sentient soul we do not experience the world passively, but approach it with our personally-tinged responses, moods and emotions. This enables us to connect with the events, things and people around us. But also with ourselves, because it is as a result of the emotions, longings and impulses of the will which are evoked in us by the world around us, that we experience ourselves in the first place. This is how we become aware of ourselves inwardly.

All the impressions and experiences which we assimilate in the course of our lives take place, in the first instance, in this sentient soul. Parts of these experiences are retained there. However, the largest part disappears deep down into the lower regions of our etheric and physical body, and thus into the unconscious regions of our soul.

The second part of the soul, the intellectual soul, enables us through logical thinking to express our experiences in words and arrange them according to their importance. This makes it possible to distinguish what is important from what is unimportant, and so we are able to make choices. Through thinking, the emotions can become true feelings. The intellectual soul stores those experiences of which we have become conscious intellectually and emotionally.

The third part of the soul is the soul of consciousness or the consciousness soul. It is the forces of this part of the soul that enable us to become conscious of the truth and the essence of things, and to understand the relationships between them. However, this works only if we come to permeate our experiences and feeling with thoughts and when we experience or feel what we think. Only then can the truth of things become apparent, and the essence become manifest. The consciousness soul contains all the truths we have taken into ourselves and of which we have become conscious.

In a previous chapter I said that our spiritual being, the spirit self, for its greatest part still lives concealed within us. Most of it lies dormant in the unconscious regions of our soul: the depths of the etheric and physical body. When however we become inwardly active, that is, turn inward in to our soul with the consciousness that comes from our higher being, it can step by step be lifted up through the different parts of the soul and so gradually awaken in the I.

First, in a more dreamy, feeling way in the sentient soul, then more clearly in concepts in the intellectual soul, until it finally becomes conscious of itself in the consciousness soul and so becomes liberated and free.[37]

When we apply this to the true conversation in which both partners show interest in each other, ask questions and listen with an active open attitude of mind to what is being told, we get the following process.

When we ask each other to speak out we recall in our sentient soul that which lives in us as feelings, questions, needs, ideas, impulses, in relation to the subject we are dealing with. That activates the soul. The experiences start to 'live' in us and we become more inwardly lively. It shows that the spirit self begins to awaken in this part of the soul. That is why so much happens already when one person gets the chance to speak with someone else who is interested, listens carefully and goes into the subject with open questions, someone who is inwardly active. When we then name the experiences that are heard, order them with the thinking and form tentative conclusions that bring us to first insights, we lift these up to the level of the intellectual soul.

A further step to an even higher level takes place in this process of awakening when we let that which we have found intellectually connect with the deeper layers of our being in the consciousness soul and let the experiences speak out their essence, their meaning.

Hans Schauder, who in his book *Conversations on Counselling* also mentions these different stages, speaks in an impressive way about the inner attitude and the quality of mind that is needed to reach this level of consciousness.[37a] He says that we should let that which we have found so far - the images of the experiences and that which we have thought about it - sink into the depths of our inner being and let them ripen there. Then after some time, answers and solutions will arise out of the depths of our soul that fill us with feelings of certainty and truth.[38]

That is how we can in true conversations help each other to awaken the higher being living in us. The insights that we receive on the level of the consciousness soul then touch us again because of their truth. We feel liberated and happy that we have found something essentially true. This emotion and happiness brings us back to our sentient soul and from there the acquired insights and truths enrich and enhance our whole soul.[39]

This is the process Rudolf Steiner refers to in his book *Occult Science* when he says that we have to raise the spirit self up from the depths of the soul through self-reflection, through our own inner activity[40]. It results in self-knowledge which is at the same time spiritual knowledge.

This reveals clearly what the process of spiritual growth entails: every time we first have to experience afresh all our experiences in the sentient soul, then we have to think about them and finally distil or 'peel' the essence out of these experiences. By repeatedly passing through this process of active self-reflection and judgement-building, the spirit being within us is gradually awakened, step by step. At the same time, this process allows us to digest the things we have experienced. Yes, there is even a close connection between the extent to which we digest our experiences and the extent to which our spiritual being is released. In his book, *Theosophy*,[41] Steiner writes: 'The human spirit grows by means of digesting the experiences.'

This spiritual growth is possible only because Christ lives in us, and when we reap the fruits of our experiences, it is he who transforms this substance of the soul into the spiritual substance of the spirit self.[42] This means that the I not only is strengthened with the power of the Spirit itself but also by the power of Christ. The same process of self-reflection and judgement-building takes place in life after death in the spiritual world. There too, we look back at our lives and experience everything afresh. The atmosphere of truth and goodness which prevails there gives us insights into all the experiences of our past life, and then we can harvest the essence of these, the fruits which it has produced. This essence is then in turn transformed into new abilities and skills with which we are born in the next life.

Now that the Spirit is becoming more active on earth, this process should also increasingly take place in our conscious life here on earth. This is the purpose of the social path. For it is only possible to harvest the fruits and the produce of our experiences on earth to the proper extent and depth, if there is another person who is willing to listen, to empathize and to think with us - a person who for a short moment is willing to serve my spiritual growth, and who in turn will need another person to help her or him go through this process her- or himself.

All this clearly shows why there is such a great need for true encounters and conversations in our time. Nowadays every person has a deep desire to be heard, seen and known. Intuitively, we are aware that we are only really born when this happens. Yet we still meet one another so little. We talk to each other about other people, work and sports, about our families and our children, but very rarely about those things which truly matter to us and which touch us inwardly.

We seem to be frightened to really respond to each other. Where will this lead to? Men, in particular, find that exploring each others' feelings or deeper needs and aims is too 'therapeutic' and prefer to avoid such situations.

But what happens in an 'official' therapeutic conversation? In fact, nothing else than that with the help of the therapist, one merely explores all sorts of experiences, or unfulfilled needs and desires which have led to problems. By going through these experiences again, thinking about them and gaining insight into them, they can be digested and assimilated and so release inner strength. Basically this inner strength is nothing other than the strength of the spirit self developing in the I. At the same time, other forces related to this process of inner growth also have an opportunity to develop. The spiritual forces which are released in this way are also used in psycho-therapy to find a new way of relating to life, and to work on the tasks which lie ahead and are necessary for development.

Thus in the end, this therapeutic process is no different from the process described before. This is because the therapist who works with experiences and insights basically follows the normal path of knowledge and insight which we must all take if we wish to understand the contents of the soul in a methodical way. Thus in fact, the therapist uses a method and social skills which we should all be mastering. It is only by developing these that we can support each other in this age of increasing chaos and despair in such a way that we provide each other with new spiritual strength.

On the other hand, it is understandable that we are anxious about true contact with other people. We are aware that in the first place, we will encounter our own impotence: the inability to be truly open to another person, to listen and respond effectively, but also to talk about what is happening inside ourselves. Both these aspects give rise to uncertainty and fear.

We become aware how difficult it is to make room for another person with true empathy and the ability to think clearly and to listen, to be open to the other as well as remaining true to oneself, to summarize the essence of what has been said, and so on. Some people are deeply shocked when they become aware how little they truly respond to others. One man who had worked on the question of the new social problems of our age for many years, told me how shocked he had been when he discovered that he was actually not at all interested in other people. He had actually never asked anyone else a question about themselves, let alone gone into this in any depth.

Conversely, meeting others can also reveal how difficult it is to show ourselves or to express what really lives in us. This is often accompanied by a great fear that other people will not respond properly. This fear is often connected with experiences during childhood and youth. Things which they had mentioned casually or in passing were used against them, or passed on to others, or misunderstood. As a result, these people became locked into themselves and so find it difficult to give themselves.

It is clear that we by nature do not possess the true social skills for the awakening of the spirit in each other. These skills must be consciously exercised and developed through trial and error. Once we have developed the correct inner attitude of respect, and are able to serve others, we gradually become aware what miracles live in true encounters.

Awakening others

Rudolf Steiner's books and lectures repeatedly contain summons to establish true social contact with other people. Particularly during the last years of his life, when the social element started to play an increasingly strong role in Anthroposophy, Steiner repeatedly stressed the importance of interest in other people, interactions on the level of the soul, and of spirit awakening encounters. He saw these activities as essential for our time:

'Despite its chaotic and tumultuous character, which will permeate our whole culture, the whole of the twentieth century will be characterized by this need – a strong need in people to be awakened by other people rather than only be awakened by the purely natural environment.' Then follow words which sound like a summons: 'The human being must become more important to his fellow human being than he has been in the past. He should become a spirit awakener for the others.' [43]

In his so-called *Letters to Members,* Rudolf Steiner frequently – and very simply – speaks about the human encounter. In the tenth letter he points out that it is often difficult for us to find words for the things that affect us most profoundly. When however there is a listener prepared to listen attentively and with respect, he says, this can loosen the other person's tongue, because it leads to trust and the possibility of finding the truth. This in turn results in a feeling of spiritual strength in the soul, where before there was impotence. It is this feeling of strength Rudolf Steiner is saying then which is what the other person is actually seeking. [44]

The next example shows how an awakening contact between human beings can work. It concerns a personal encounter of myself with a boy who was thirteen years old. The boy asked me to talk with him about life and about the world. I felt that he did not so much expect any answers from me, as that he wanted to formulate his own ideas. Therefore I refrained from giving answers and adopted a more questioning approach going into that which he brought forward. Then I tried to raise what he told me to a higher insight and relate it to other matters. Amazingly this joint process resulted in the boy gaining more and more insights himself: insights into life, into the human I, and the social tasks of our time which revealed great wisdom.

During this dialogue, which took place while we were walking, he stood still at a certain moment and said: 'You know, I feel so free.' A little later he put his hands round his head and said: 'Oh, I'm so glad that I am able to think.'

During our second talk I asked the boy why he thought he was able to express such wise words on subjects which had surely never been mentioned at home or at school. He gave me the following answer: 'You know, I'm just an ordinary boy, but when you speak with me like this, I become liberated.' When I asked him how he thought this happens, he said: 'There is a door inside us. That door is in your feelings, but it is locked. When you talk to me like this, the door opens and then I am freed and can say things, I don't know where they come from. Then I feel happy and strong.'

What happened in our dialogues? By listening to him and asking him questions, cautiously broadening the answers and looking for the essence, the boy's higher self was gradually awakened. This process took place because a connection was made between his ordinary I (ego) 'I'm just an ordinary boy' and the higher or spirit self, both that working from the inside, and that working from the outside.

The experience of the liberating effect of his higher self then makes him say: 'I feel so free.' Immediately afterwards, the boy says: 'Oh, I'm so glad that I can think.' This means that he felt grateful - to a large extent, unconsciously - that the creative force of the Spirit was working in his thinking, enabling him to gain insights into things. It is gratitude towards that part of the spirit self which works from the outside via his thinking in his I. This is shown by the gesture of taking his head into his hands.

Our second conversation led to the answer to my question of where all these wise insights came from. 'I'm just an ordinary boy, but when you talk with me like this, it's as though I'm liberated.' With these words he refers to his inner spirit self. This is also evident from the fact that he points to the soul, where the 'I' is hidden behind the locked door. The door can open when another person relates to him in a particular way, resulting in an inner event. It is this inner I or spirit self, he then says, that enables him to say things, although he does not know where they come from.

Like the experience of the group described in a previous chapter, this experience results in a special after-feeling: strength and happiness. The connection which is forged for a while between the boy's ordinary I and the spiritual world allows some of the strength and happiness which are part of that world to flow directly into him.

Finally, the boy's modesty and simplicity about his insights and experiences are quite remarkable.

This example clearly shows that the world of the spirit is real. It shows that there is truth in the anthroposophical idea that a higher self exists in the deeper regions of the soul, a self which is infinitely greater and stronger than our ordinary ego, with a consciousness with which our ordinary daily consciousness completely pales in comparison. This higher self can be freed thanks to the awakening effect that is possible between the soul and spirit of one person and the other. In what happens *between human beings*, Rudolf Steiner says, we can perceive what the spiritual world really is. At the same time, it enables us to understand the essence of Anthroposophy. Anthroposophy is not a theoretical spiritual science; but is essentially a living spiritual experience.

Steiner formulates this as follows: 'We may assimilate all sorts of wonderful anthroposophical ideas from this knowledge of the spiritual world, we can theoretically understand everything that is said about the etheric and the astral body and so on, but this does not mean that we understand the spiritual world. We start to develop an understanding of the spiritual world only when we wake up to the inner being or spirit self of the other person. Only then, can there be a true understanding of Anthroposophy.'[45]

Of course, this does not mean that we do not need the insights and 'ideas' of Anthroposophy. We certainly do need them to shed light on our personal experiences. However, we should not keep them in our head as abstract theories, but they should become practically active in the soul, there where in our own time the spiritual being wants to awaken.

The liberating insight

By means of these stimulating and spirit awakening conversations, we connect each other with the spirit self which exists in the soul. This is only possible because in these encounters consciousness is generated through inner activity, or in other words, because a process of spiritual insight takes place. We will take a closer look at the essential steps in this process and will see where they lead to.

The first step towards the spirit in our own inner self starts with the experience of things in our own sentient soul. As we saw above, we need each other's help to do this. By listening and asking questions, we must help the other person in such a way that the memories of earlier experiences are reawakened and can be experienced again. At the same time, the longings, ideals and impulses in the soul related to what is yet to develop, must also be awakened. In this way it is as though the past and the future come closer together.

All these thoughts, experiences, longings and ideals which reside in the soul are connected with a multitude of emotions, fears, sorrows and pain, as well as with pleasure and enthusiasm. This is why, as soon as they arise in a conversation, they result in inner movement in that person. This leads to the first essential connection of the I with the inner spirit self. This essential connection does not take place when this stage is omitted, and the other person talks about her- or himself in a rather abstract, distant or impersonal way. In that case, nothing happens. This is because the connection point of the inner spirit self in the soul lies in the region of experiences, desires and emotions and below that. This region is part of the sentient soul, and not part of the intellectual soul. Therefore the stage of connecting with the experiences and feelings is actually the most important stage in the process of self-knowledge, and in the connection with our inner self. If we are for any reason unable to connect properly with our experiences and emotions, we will *not* be able to establish a true connection with our spirit self!

In the next stage of the process, we ask questions with our thinking about all these experiences, starting with more details and facts, which can clarify matters and make them more specific. This results in a sense of order in the soul. We think about what we have experienced and reach provisional conclusions. This means that the process of knowledge has progressed by another step, so that we can distinguish between what is important and what is unimportant. It provides a first insight into things, but is still predominantly an intellectual, rational insight. We may know a few things, but at this level, we do not understand their true meaning. To do this, we have to take another step, now to the level of the spirit.

This step starts with the following question: I may have made such and such a discovery or gained such and such an insight, but what does it really mean? Or what is the essence of these things? Or what is really being said?

We will only find an answer to these questions if we take them inside ourselves and put them to our spirit self. To do this, it is as though we have to 'open up' the question inwardly, without giving any answers ourselves, and then let it go, so that it disappears entirely for a moment. By letting it go, we go through a point where for a while we really do not know anything anymore. When this happens, an answer can suddenly spring up from the inner spirit self, and this contains a truth, the essence of the perception concerned. In the chapter, *Light in the Soul*, I mentioned how well Hans Schauder described the inner attitude belonging to this process in his book *Conversations on Counselling*. How can this process towards spiritual insight be applied in ordinary daily life? An example may show this.

Once, when my car broke down, I drove home with the driver of the breakdown truck who was taking me and my car home. We started talking about his work and his everyday life. I asked him many questions about his experiences, and we carefully came to some insights. At a certain point I asked him: 'What is the most important aspect of your work for you?' He was quiet for a moment, and then he said: 'The fact that I become aware of the relative nature of existence: people leave home in the morning, but don't know what experiences they'll have that day. Some don't even come back home.'

It was clear that with these words my driver was saying something essential about himself and his experiences in life, although he had never been aware of these in this way before.

This happened because he had taken my questions inside his conscious soul, and was going through all the experiences we had discussed with his feelings and his thoughts. Then he let them go for a moment and then the answer came from deep within: 'that I become aware of the relative nature of existence.'

However, such an essential idea expressed in such terms connected to the self, can be obtained only if we do not think intellectually about the questions raised, or speculate or fantasize about its possible meaning, because then we do not let go of the level of consciousness of our ordinary personality and the intellectual soul. We have to go to the level of the spirit, and this is possible only if we let go of the insight discovered by ordinary thinking, so that it can open up within us and dissolve into nothingness for a moment. When we reach this level, the spirit which lives in our inner self can rearrange all the perceptions in a new way and express them afresh.[45] This results in insights which are not purely intellectual or speculative, but which express a truth. In this case: 'that I become aware of the relative nature of existence.'

How can we know that the truths we have discovered are real truths and not illusions? How do we experience that something is true? We do this with an inner 'knowledge', which at the same time is an experience of knowledge and a knowing experience. This is a quality of our own inner spirit self. The truth we discover at this level is accompanied by a feeling of evidence; henceforth it is an incontrovertible truth for us.

Anyone who, while seeking for truth, has penetrated the level of the spirit, has thus reached a level which at the same time is both deeply personal and objective. This is why we are able to share the truth we have found with other people on this level, and can truly understand each other here. The truth, which the driver of the breakdown truck discovered in our encounter, also comes across as a truth to me. In this case, it was he who discovered the essence of his experience, but it could also have been I who discovered it. If I had taken the experiences of this man inside me, and had formed an accurate inner picture of them, this truth would also have appeared in me. If I had then returned the truth I had discovered to him, he would also have recognized himself in it.

Such encounters are fruitful for both partners, even if the contribution of one is more geared to listening and asking, while that of the other is more geared to talking. In both encounters I have described, it was not only my partner who was linked more closely to his spirit self, but my own spirit self was also addressed when I listened actively and thought with him. After all, I assimilated something of the content of my partner's soul into my own soul. I did this by experiencing within myself what was alive in the other person, by reflecting on it and raising it to the level of the spirit. Through this my own spirit self was also awakened. As Rudolf Steiner said: 'The perception of oneself,' i.e., of that which forms the content of the soul, even if these are the experiences of someone else - 'is at the same time an awakening of the Self.' [46] This is what I experience when after a good conversation I feel more strength, harmony and inner richness in myself, even if I was mainly listening. This leads us to the conclusion that:

When I succeed in completing the process of spiritual insight in a conversation to the level of the consciousness-soul and the spirit, I am raising both the other person and myself to a higher spiritual level.

This true process of spiritual knowledge, which brings about spiritual awakening, is not only important for human beings, but is also important for the world of nature. For we human beings have the task not only to awaken the forces of the spirit in our fellow human beings, but also in our fellow creatures in the world of the minerals, the plants, the trees and the animals. This we do if we do not simply look around in the world of nature in a superficial way, but if we take such a deep interest in all these creatures that we experience something of their essence and learn to know their spiritual being through their shapes, colours and style of growth. In fact the same method can be used here as I described before in the spirit awakening process of the human being. We, for instance, observe a certain plant or animal, let these perceptions come to 'life', to live, in our sentient soul by feeling and experiencing it, then observe it more factually and in greater detail with our intellectual soul and finally let it speak out its inner essence in our consciousness soul and spirit. Rudolf Steiner describes this path very beautifully in the first chapter of his book *How to Know Higher Worlds.* [47]

By doing this, we start to liberate the spiritual beings in the plants, trees and nature from the spell, their imprisonment in physical matter, and thus also from the grasp of the counter-forces. In the words of Rudolf Steiner:

'A person who has acquired insight is not an inactive observer of the universe around him who conjures up images of something which would also exist without him. The strength of his knowledge is a higher force, a creative natural force. That which flashes up in him is something divine which was under a spell before, and which would lie fallow without his search for insight, to await another liberator. Thus the human personality does not live in itself and for itself; it lives for the world.' [47A]

Two thousand years ago, the apostle Paul already beautifully formulated this liberating task of mankind as regards creation. In his letter to the Romans, he wrote, after emphasizing the fact that we are heirs of God and co-heirs of Christ:

For the earnest expectation of the creature waiteth for the manifestation of the sons of God. [48]

For the creature was made subject to vanity, not willingly, but by reason of him who hath subjected the same in hope.

Because the creature itself also shall be delivered from the bondage of corruption into the glorious liberty of the children of God.

For we know that the whole creation groaneth and travaileth in pain together until now. And not only they, but ourselves also, which have the first fruits of the Spirit, even we ourselves groan within ourselves, waiting for the adoption, to wit, the redemption of our body.

It depends on our spiritual efforts and loving interest whether the spirit can be redeemed and liberated from the forces of evil in the world of the Father, which is falling apart. However, it is not our 'ordinary' personality which achieves this redemption, it is the Spirit, behind which stands the living Christ and which can work through us because of our inner activity. It is only the divine aspect in us that can liberate the divine aspects in nature and in other people.

Michael

When we human beings truly acquire a knowledge of the essence of living creatures, we contribute to their redemption and their liberation from the grasp of the counterforces. Then the divine-spiritual element which once radiated from the Divine Trinity as a living reality to become imprisoned in the physical forms of creation, can be liberated and continue to develop to higher levels. If we wish to take on this task with regard to creation, we must develop our capacity for knowledge which has been trained by external reality so that it becomes clear and receptive to the inner, spiritual reality of things. When we do this, trying to develop our knowledge and understanding in this way, we form a connection with the Spirit of the time, Michael – whether we are aware of this or not.

Michael is the Christian name of a high divine being from the ranks of the divine hierarchies, the different groups of spiritual beings which are above mankind, and are represented at the lowest level by the angels. These spiritual beings direct the development of the earth and mankind in the service of the Divine Trinity. In our own time, when we are increasingly confronted with the forces of evil, Michael is the leading spirit of the time, or archè. This means that in our time, he leads the divine hierarchies and human development on earth. His aim is to restrict the power of evil, and to help people connect with the world of the spirit.

In addition to being the leading spirit of our time, Michael has traditionally been the lord of the forces of intelligence in the cosmos. What does this mean?

We have seen how essential our thinking capacity is for the connection with the world of the spirit, and for our own development and that of others. The field of the intellect, of perception and conceptual thought is basically the only way in which we, as people of the earth, still have a direct and open connection with our spirit self, and therefore with the spiritual world. This intellect or capacity for thinking was granted us by God so that we could become free, independent individuals. It is the capacity for independent thinking, in interacting with the spirit outside us, that allows us to develop our inner spiritual being and consciousness.

Once, the human intellect formed part of the cosmic intelligence which operates in the divine-spiritual world. In his *Leading Thoughts*,[49] Rudolf Steiner used grand images to describe what this cosmic intelligence entailed. In earthly terms it can be conceived as powerful images of thought which constantly create new realities. The divine being which is responsible for the proper management of this creative world of thoughts is Michael.

In the course of evolution, cosmic intelligence, cosmic thinking has increasingly become incarnated in mankind. It is possible to follow this incarnation of thinking step-by-step, by seeing how philosophy has developed through the ages.[50] The more this cosmic thinking incarnated in individuals, resulting in individualised thinking, the more it became separated from the divine creative forces it originated from and became increasingly dead and abstract. This was a necessary process. Inwardly, in our thinking, we human beings had to break away from the living wisdom and full richness of the divine beings which had determined our will and our feelings, and filled our thoughts since the beginnings of time. It was only in this way that we could develop the activity of thinking and knowledge through our own efforts, and so could develop our I and in that our inner spirit self. If we had not been able to separate away from the divine world in our thinking, this would not have been possible. That is why the whole tragedy of the process of separation from the divine world had to take place. The lonely life and the bareness of earthly existence has a profound meaning and significance. After all, it is only because our thinking has lost all living spiritual strength that we can move freely in them. It is only in the medium of a dead, earthly way of thinking that we are truly free, and that we can learn how to use this freedom ourselves.

Rudolf Steiner expressed this as follows:

> 'These thoughts, which are the entire basis of human freedom, do not force us precisely because they are dead, because they are not alive. Nowadays, we can become free creatures, because we are not concerned with living, but with dead thoughts. We can pick up these dead thoughts and use them freely.'[51]

It is actually this lifeless thinking which can grant us living freedom – and not only freedom, but also a new connection with the spiritual world, now through our inner being, the divine aspect *inside* us. This freedom is at the same time the essential condition for the fortifying, healing encounter with Christ in our time. During the present stage of development we can only connect with him – and with the other spiritual forces which help us – in a state of freedom. It is only if we take the step ourselves that we can join forces with the inner strength of Christ. I will return to this aspect of the connection with Christ later on.

However, as the intellect became more abstract, the counter-forces were also able to extend their influence in human beings. This applied particularly to Ahriman, who is the great inspirator of abstract thinking. As a result of his influence, the last remnants of the ability to think in true, living images disappeared during the course of the nineteenth century. Abstract thought cannot conceive in any way the spiritual processes and forces which are active in the external world. Our present science and culture were produced by these abstract thoughts. They have given us external freedom, and enormous material strength, but they face life uncomprehendingly and with empty hands – both our own life and that of the whole of creation. With this dead thinking, we have arrived at a zero point in our human evolution.

Michael's task is now to connect this capacity of thinking, which is so essential for our human development, again to the divine world. However, he can fulfil this task only if we become inwardly active ourselves. In other words, if we once again connect our thinking with the cosmic intelligence entrusted to Michael. How can we ensure that Michael is able to save our thinking, which has already fallen so wholly into the power of Ahriman? How can this be done?

In fact, it is possible because Christ connected with mankind and the earth up to the level of the physical, two thousand years ago, thus descending into the realm of Ahriman. He brought to it an intelligence which was equivalent to the original divine spiritual force of creation, the force which once created the cosmos and everything in it. This force is the Logos, the creative Word which once created heaven, earth, mankind and the natural world, and which lives among us and in our souls since the events of Golgotha.[52]

Since that time, two sorts of intelligence have acted within us: one which is mastered by Ahriman, and one which contains the Logos force of Christ. This enables us to make choices. If we do not make a choice, and do not take responsibility for our own way of thinking, the Ahrimanic style of thinking will continue to grow within us.

The thinking connected with Christ can develop only if we wish this ourselves and are prepared to develop a new way of thinking. This must be a style of thinking in which we in a lively way, form in ourselves images of the processes of spiritual development which are active in mankind, in nature and in the cosmos as I described before. This means that we should not deal with our observations and experiences in a vague, emotional way, because this would take us into imaginary, illusory realms, and thus straight into the arms of the other counter-force: Lucifer. Thinking in the sense of the intelligence of Christ means, in the first place, talking about nature and mankind in the way that is usual in scientific thought.[53] This means that we must be able to think about things in the world in a clear, logical, factual way. This is the first step. Then we should go a level deeper and learn to know and understand the spiritual processes living in mankind and in nature by means of the intuitive process of knowledge and empathy which I have referred to before. This means that we must learn to 'read' the external appearance of a tree, a plant, an animal or a human being, and their development in time, as expressions of inner spiritual forces, forces with an inner life. This means that eventually the essence of what is observed can manifest itself.

Acquiring insight in this way means gaining an insight into the meaning of the Christ intelligence. In this way the force of the Word, the Logos, which lives within us, and which we can also call the force of the Holy Spirit sent by Christ, can become active. This is what liberates the spiritual forces imprisoned in mankind and nature *through us*. Rudolf Steiner described this process of liberation as follows:

'However, if we allow Christ to accompany us, if we take our dead thoughts with him into the world of the stars, if we take them into the world of the sun and the moon, of clouds, mountains and rivers, of minerals, plants and animals, if we take them into the whole of the physical human world, then everything we observe in nature will become alive, and the Holy Spirit, the living, healing spirit which resurrects us from death, will rise up as from the grave from all creatures. Then we will feel that, accompanied by Christ, we have been given new life from that which was experienced as death. We can feel the living, healing spirit in all the creatures of this world, speaking to us.' [54]

This is the task and the process the apostle Paul was talking about in his letter to the Romans. It is by developing the Christ intelligence within us that we turn our abstract thinking back into a spiritual organ of knowledge, and so return it to Michael. In this way we are acting and fighting with Michael for the light and for the progress of humanity, nature and the earth.

The more we connect with Michael in this way, the more Christ can become active in the creation of the Father through our intuitive, understanding consciousness, so that he can liberate the living spirit concealed in this. This happens every time when a human being consciously performs a creative act of knowledge and love. In this way, the spirit of Christ which is active within us gradually transforms the transient world of the Father, step by step, into the eternal substance of his Spirit. This will continue until there is a new heaven, a new earth and a new mankind in which the Divine Trinity will manifest in an entirely new way.

Self-knowledge and change

The day-to-day practice

The previous chapters revealed an aspect of the social ideal of our human development and of the tremendous task we have in relation to our fellow human beings. This is why Rudolf Steiner said: 'Our task, the most important task we have for the future, is wanting to learn to understand people.' [55]

We may well ask why this task, understanding people, is so difficult. Why do we do so many things with each other, and yet remain so unprepared to really know one another?

Of course, we are aware that understanding other people and relating to them is essential. The problems which we all have in our relationships with other people clearly show this. But at the same time we also feel that this process requires a great deal of effort and energy. This goes against our nature. Subconsciously, we know that we need to go through an intense process of inner change and development when we truly want to meet the other person. We not only have to empathize and think with that other person, we must also be able to experience that which lives in the other in ourselves. In other words, we must feel this inwardly and bring this to life in our own soul. This is certainly not a self-evident skill, but something which we must learn and achieve through our own efforts.

Secondly, we should not only be able to follow the thoughts of the other person, but should also actively think ourselves, and search for insight. This does not happen automatically either. Finally, we should also master the ability to grasp the essence of things. In other words, we should learn to perform a process of true judgement-building, of true insight into another person, starting on the level of the experiences and leading to the level of the spirit.

This process however is only possible when we get true insight into ourselves, true self-knowledge. By self-knowledge, I mean acquiring an insight into our own way of thinking, feeling, experiencing and acting, and thus into our place in the world and the way in which we relate to other people. If we are completely honest about this, we will come to the conclusion that in the way we usually think, feel and act, we do not perceive the other person at all, let alone understand him or her as he/she really is. We then see that all our soul qualities are nowadays totally focused on ourselves and on our subjective experiences and perceptions, and very very little or not at all on the other human being as such. Taking one step further in our process of self-knowledge, we will become aware that in our communication with others, all sorts of unconscious opinions, habits, sympathies and antipathies, aversions, undigested aggressions and so on, play a role. In other words, we not only perceive very little about other people, but in addition, we colour what we do perceive, transforming it in accordance with our own preferences and prejudices. This then forms the basis of our relationship, and it is with this inaccurate image of the other person that we enter into a 'dialogue' with her or him.

It is very important to understand that this sort of approach does not leave the other person unaffected. It results in the other in more than an awareness of not being able to relate, or of not being understood. If I approach a colleague on the basis of an untrue or rigid image, this really affects him or her. For if he does not understand that situation, he will become imprisoned, both in himself and in his relationship with me. This is the reason why people in relationships so often 'close up' inwardly, or become impotently furious without knowing why. This is the opposite of what happens in a true encounter. If, in the contact with another person, we succeed in developing an aspect of truth about him or her, we help that person to liberate some of his or her spirit self. If we develop untruth, we imprison the other person in her- or himself as well as our relationship.

The above gives a clear picture of the effect of Ahriman. If we do not start a real process of attaining consciousness in our own soul when we are in contact with another person, this counter-force takes the chance to oppress the other person, imprison him in himself and obstruct his development and our relationship.

It is only when we have the courage to look at these facts which always play a part in our relationships with other people, and when we experience them in our own soul as a shocking truth, that we will be ready for change and prepared to take the first steps towards a real encounter.

The rhythm of the soul

Why is our nature so disinclined to learn about the being of others? We can only discover the answer to this question if we gain a greater insight into the operation of the soul. To do this, we will have to take another little detour.

Our soul is characterized by a great deal of movement. This movement is caused by two opposing forces which are the foundation of our whole psychological life. One force enables us to move out of ourselves so that we can connect with the world around us. The other force separates us from the world, pulling us back inside into our own inner world. The first happens for instance when we are breathlessly listening to music in the concert hall: we become separated from ourselves and lose ourselves in the music, becoming one with it. The second thing happens when we are distracted by something: in the row in front of us somebody may be moving their head in time to the music. The whole top half of their body seems to be moving. This can cause a slight irritation. At that moment we are back inside ourselves, and the world is separate from us, confronting us.

In Anthroposophy, these basic gestures of the soul – this primordial rhythm of connecting and separating, of opening up and contracting – are known as the movements of sympathy and antipathy. These terms are used in an entirely neutral way; sympathy is not 'good', and antipathy is not 'bad'. The movement of sympathy in the soul connects us with the world around us, removing us from ourselves. The movement of antipathy frees us from the world around us, so that we return into ourselves. Both movements are necessary for a healthy development of our personality and a healthy interaction with the outside world. In Anthroposophy sympathy and antipathy are related to the processes of falling asleep and waking up. This indicates that these movements are also linked to changes in consciousness. Each time it flows into the outside world, our self-consciousness momentarily descends to the level of sleep. When it contracts, the soul awakens and comes to itself.

This movement of falling asleep and waking up, of sympathy and antipathy, of connection and separation, developed when the human spirit separated away from the divine world to go its own way. Once it lived in the enormous and all-encompassing atmosphere of sympathy in the harmony, bliss and undivided unity of the divine world. There was no separation in this heavenly atmosphere, and therefore there was no self-consciousness. This could develop only when the original human spirit separated from the divine world, went its own way and developed its own thinking and consciousness, thanks to the gifts of the beings of the divine world.

The rhythm of connecting and contracting, of surrender and separation, which we find at every level of our life, evolved in the polarity between the developing individual human spirit and the divine world. It is reflected in the great rhythm of death and birth; in other words, of excarnation and incarnation. It is reflected in the alternating pattern of sleep and wakefulness, day and night, and in the process of 'sleeping into' things around us and waking up in ourselves. This polarity is found even in the process of the acquisition of knowledge. Every perception takes us for a moment into the object outside, while the concept, the thinking about this object, takes us back into our self.

Our self-consciousness develops in all these thousands of movements to and fro between falling asleep and waking up, between sympathy and antipathy, which we make every day at every level of life. For example, if I enjoy a beautiful sunset in the evening, I will in the first instance, 'sleep into' this observation, losing the consciousness of myself as a separate person. Then I feel a need stirring to find myself again.

I withdraw and become aware of my own enjoyment. This *makes me aware* of my enjoyment, and I become conscious that it is I who am experiencing the beauty around me.

As I wrote in an earlier chapter, our own consciousness develops very gradually from the depths of the soul upwards. In the first instance, it still lives as a deep unconsciousness at the lowest levels of the soul. It is asleep in our instincts and passions, it becomes gradually more distinct in our experiences, clearer in our intellectual thinking, and truly clearly conscious at the level of the consciousness-soul and the spirit, where we can grasp essential and objective truths. Our consciousness actually consists of a complex of different degrees of consciousness taken from the different layers of the soul. The brighter our consciousness shines, the stronger our self-awareness, and thus our experience of our self as an independent personality.

The basic rhythm of sympathy and antipathy described above operates at every layer of the soul. Therefore an understanding of this rhythm of the soul is an essential instrument for our personal developmental path towards the spirit.

The 'basic social phenomenon'

All these aspects play a role in our contacts with other people, making the interaction between people extremely complicated. Not only is there a constant process of 'sleeping into and waking up', taking place in each of us personally at every level of our life and soul, but this same process also takes place in our interaction with each other.

What happens when two human beings stand opposite each other? Rudolf Steiner described this as follows: 'When two human beings stand opposite each other, one is always trying to put the other person to sleep, while the other is always trying to stay awake. This is ... the basic phenomenon in social science.' [56] When I stand opposite another person, my attention is momentarily caught by him or her, and for a moment I lose consciousness of myself, just as with everything else I observe in the outside world. It is as though the other person hypnotizes me for a moment, putting me to 'sleep'. Then the sense of survival and the feeling of self reassert themselves and I return to myself. In this process it is as though we are vibrating between sleeping into the other person, waking up in ourselves, sleeping again into the other person, and waking up again in our own consciousness. This is a constant process when we are in contact with another person. We do not know that it is happening, because it takes place in the unconscious regions of the will.[57]

At the point that I sleep into the other and my self-consciousness is reduced to the level of unconsciousness, my soul flows into the world of the other person's experiences and soul, and assimilates an element of this.[58] I am not conscious of what I take in from that other person's world of experience, because I am 'sleeping' there. For the

brief moment that my soul becomes so immersed in the
other person's soul, we are unified in a social gesture, connected together in 'sympathy'. However, I am afraid of
losing my self-consciousness altogether if I remain 'asleep'
in the other person for too long, and therefore there is a
movement of antipathy: I withdraw and become conscious
of myself again. My soul closes up, the connection is
broken, and we stand opposite each other once again as two
separate persons. The same process also takes place in the
other person in a corresponding fashion. This is why Steiner
says that when two people stand opposite each other, one is
trying to put the other to sleep, while the other tries to
remain awake. However, this unconscious interaction actually changes both. Because afterwards an aspect of the
other person now lives in me and an aspect of me lives in the
other person, neither of us is the same person that he or she
was before.

Steiner calls this tendency to sleep into the other person
by losing the consciousness of oneself and being assimilated
by the other person, the social impulse. In this context he
means the force of sympathy which connects us to the other
person in a reflex action. Thanks to this force we human
beings who become increasingly separated from each other
as individuals, can lose our self-consciousness for a moment
and enter the soul and the being of the other person. This
brings us briefly to the unconscious state of unity which was
characteristic of our togetherness in the divine world in the
past.

Steiner calls the other force which pulls us back into
ourselves with a gesture of antipathy, the antisocial impulse,
because it breaks the unconscious connection with the other
person, so that we once again stand opposite him or her as
a separate individual. The antisocial impulse springs from
our own intellectual abilities and consciousness, and is
therefore related to the development of the I-personality
and self-consciousness. Because we are thinking people, we

are antisocial, i.e., we are able to look at the world around us without losing ourselves in it.[59]

If we did not have our own individual thinking and self-consciousness, we human beings would immediately be returned to the unconscious state of primordial interconnection. Therefore this situation is immediately restored at times when our own consciousness is extinguished, as it is in sleep during the night, or in life after death. As Rudolf Steiner says:

'In this state (...) it is possible unconsciously to build the bridge connecting us with all people.' But he continues to say that even when we are awake, '(...) the other person opposite us wishes to unconsciously put us to sleep so that the bridge can be built to him - and we do the same to him. But we must guard against this, because otherwise we would be deprived of our thinking consciousness in our relationship with people.' That is why – subconsciously – every person is a threat to our own thinking, and we are inclined to protect our thoughts from the other, and that is why 'we are highly antisocial beings as regards our thinking (...)' [60]

As I said above, this vibration between sleeping into the other person and waking up in ourselves takes place in the unconscious area of the will. However, it can also be found in a more conscious area, for instance, in a conversation. I 'enter into' another person when I listen to him or her as a result of the effect of the social impulse. If however I do this by returning to myself momentarily from time to time while I am listening, and then returning to the other person again the next moment, I will not lose myself entirely in that other person, and then I do become conscious of what is going on in him or her. However, I will only be able to express this at the point at which the antisocial impulse brings me back to myself again, and when I am able to think about what I have perceived and experienced. If I then give the other person my response, he or she in turn will sleep into me as a result of the social impulse, and so on. This shows that the 'toing and froing' between the other person and myself is actually the basic phenomenon of social life.

In fact these impulses are in constant conflict with each other, both in ourselves and in our relationships with other people. One part of us wishes to lose itself in the other person, thus wishing to become part again of the primordial state of unconscious belonging, and to forget the pain of separation and loneliness. Another part of us, which is related to our I and our independence as an individual, however, rejects this utterly. In fact, that part of us wishes to keep other people outside us as far as possible, and even wants to push them away. The antisocial impulse becomes stronger the more our intellectual capacities and our I and personality are powerfully developed. People in whom the antisocial impulse is not so strong therefore find it easier 'to sleep in' into other people. It is still natural for their souls to flow into the souls of others. On the other hand, these people have little consciousness of themselves as a separate person. What problems arise when these two different sorts of people are in a relationship together is something everyone may have experienced already.

In an age when the consciousness soul, and thus self-consciousness, must develop, the antisocial impulses will become stronger and stronger. This means that people are becoming increasingly locked up in themselves, increasingly face each other as strangers, and have the greatest trouble in reaching and understanding each other. At the same time, they become less able to connect with others in the old, unconscious way. Obviously all this will result in an enormous sense of loneliness and loss. As this situation gets worse this means also that the clashes, conflicts and wars between people will increase.

Working on the encounter
with other people

The antisocial impulse means that people feel the need not to lose themselves in their contact with other people, but in fact to face other people, measuring up to them. This drive is even greater when the person has a powerful personality as a result of a well-developed intellect or strong will. This means that we who predominantly have this force constantly want to be the strongest, the most intelligent, the wittiest; in other words, to be one up on the other person. The need for contact is suppressed, but usually resurfaces in a rather distorted way on another plane.

The other extreme surfaces when, because of the predominance of the sympathetic force, and the wish to experience our connection with the other strongly, we merge into the other person to such an extent that we lose ourselves. This need means that we suppress parts of ourselves which do not fit into this harmony or connection, and pretend that they do not exist. But usually they will reappear in a different way and in a distorted form again.

As I said before: these two tendencies are found at every layer of consciousness in the soul, and therefore also in our thinking, feeling and in the will. They are there because they belong to our ordinary personality and are therefore 'natural'. The soulforces in our time are only directed towards ourselves and our own needs and development. This has to do with the development of our own personality and I. Thus they prevent us from achieving a true encounter with another person. Instead of learning to know the other person, these tendencies actually shut us off from each other. The other person her- or himself is not the aim of the contact, but the means I can use to become more myself, or to experience myself in a particular way. Unconsciously my attitude to the other person is: what have you got which could be useful to me? Or: in what way do you threaten my sense of self, my independence, the realization of my self?

How do these antisocial impulses work in us at the different levels of the soul in our contact with other people? How do they create openings for the effects of counter-forces?

In *thinking,* the antisocial gesture is expressed in the fact that we stay in ourselves and do not take the step towards the inner being of the other person to immerse ourselves in him or her. That is because basically we are not interested in the being of the other, in the thoughts, the experiences and the motives of the other person. Our own thoughts and views are the most important thing. Often, we will openly reveal hidden criticisms of what the other person is saying, or the way in which he or she is saying it. We prefer speaking to listening. This leads to a tendency to state our own view of everything the other person says. Thus we clearly show or imply what the other person is doing wrong, or how he or she is mistaken. The views which are expressed often contain a moral judgment of the other person. This attitude is so antisocial because it actually makes it impossible for the other person to express himself. Instead of being liberated and being encouraged to speak, he is shut in and unable to express himself. In this case, we see that the thinking process is used above all as a means of experiencing oneself and maintaining one's own identity in relation to the other person. When this is accompanied by criticism and moral judgements, there is also an exercising of power. Thus we see here the force of Ahriman at work, which imprisons the other person by means of negative, oppressive thoughts and a critical approach.

In the field of *feeling,* the forces of antipathy and sympathy reveal themselves in conversation. If, in the person who is listening, there is a predominant feeling of antipathy towards the person who is talking, her or his soul will be largely shut off from the other person in an antisocial gesture. The other person will not find the space in which to express her- or himself, but meets resistance. In some cases the person who is talking gradually becomes aware of the other person's feelings of antipathy during the conversation. She or he senses that what she or he says is being distorted by the other person, and is misunderstood or ignored, so that saying what there is to say becomes increasingly difficult and strained.

Obviously there can be all sorts of more or less understandable 'reasons' for these feelings of antipathy. Often they are merely unconscious prejudices or associations with negative experiences in the past. However, it may also happen that the person who is listening is afraid to be taken over by the other person, or by what he is saying, and of losing her- or himself in this. In this case, people evoke feelings of antipathy in themselves to maintain their identity vis-à-vis the other person. Of course, this happens unconsciously. When asked where the antipathy comes from, they will hardly be able to give a clear answer.

Thus in our feelings of antipathy we are primarily maintaining our identity vis-à-vis the other person, and so become conscious of ourselves. This is why the feeling of antipathy is often pleasurable. We feel a sense of power over the other person, particularly if it is someone who is happy to merge into us, and we can push him away with this attitude of antipathy.

The situation is completely different when the feeling of sympathy is predominant. Our feelings of sympathy can be so strong that we completely lose ourselves in the person who is talking, or who fascinates us, or by the compelling character of her or his story. We are unable to maintain our own thinking activity, and flow into the other person, losing ourselves, our self-consciousness, in her or him. The result is that we are not able to reproduce what she or he has said very well, and are unable to respond to it.

Nevertheless, someone who listens in this way can have the feeling that she or he is a very good sounding board for the other person, and is therefore acting in a very social way. After all, the other person has been able to say what she or he wanted to say, and enjoyed the attention it received. In reality, we did create a space for the other person to express himself, but while he was talking, we were more focused on the feelings it aroused in us than trying to understand the other person through what he was saying.

Of course, in itself there is no objection to people losing themselves in each other. It can be necessary and very pleasant. However, it is not correct to describe this process as truly social. A truly social interaction occurs only if the contact is not used primarily for us to experience ourselves, but if it is used to really get to know the other person. If he is truly seeking contact, he will feel left in the cold by my selfish way of listening. He will feel – even if only unconsciously – that he is only important to me in so far as I can experience something of myself through him, and that he will be forgotten moments later.

People who lose themselves in the feelings and experiences of contact with another person often confuse this feeling with love. Rudolf Steiner described this mistake in strong terms: 'A person imagines that he loves someone, but in this love he actually loves only himself. This is a source of antisocial behaviour which can, moreover, be the source of terrible self-deception. For example, we may imagine that we are overflowing with love for someone, while in fact we do not love that other person, but we love being connected to the other person in our own soul (...) This is an important secret of life. It is incredibly important, because the misconception about this love which we see as love, but which is actually only self-love, selfishness and self-interest, and by far the majority of love which exists between people and is described as love is mere egoism in disguise - this misconception is the source of the greatest, most widespread antisocial impulses. Self-love parading as love turns man into an antisocial creature in the strongest sense.' [61]

The effect of the counter-forces can also be identified in the one-sided domination of the forces of antipathy or the forces of sympathy in our feelings. Ahriman's influence can be seen in the feelings of antipathy which always contain some measure of hatred towards the other person, and also in the mockery or cynicism which accompanies the experience of one's own power and the vulnerability of the other person. Lucifer's influence is apparent when someone cherishes his own feelings in the contact with the other person, without a moment's concern for that other person. Usually Ahriman and Lucifer work together at this level, and if we are not sufficiently self-aware, we can be thrown back and forth between the two. For example, we can be strongly attracted to someone and get a great deal out of the contact, until that person says or does something which evokes an angry response. Then the pendulum swings to the other side, the side of Ahriman. The dream is suddenly broken and the relationship no longer produces delightful feelings. We have a sense of being cheated, and in many cases this leads to hatred and aggression, and the need to hurt the other person.

The antisocial conduct in the field of *the will and behaviour* is expressed in the tendency to acknowledge what the other person says or is, only if it accords with our own views, feelings or habits, and to deny or undermine, mock or punish everything which deviates from this. In this way, we not only put our own stamp on that person, but also force him away from himself. In this way an essential aspect of the being of that other person is affected or smothered at source.

Where does this antisocial attitude come from? In the first place, it comes from the need to express ourselves in the world, creating a space for ourselves. But we do this in such a way that we cross over the boundaries of other people's identities as though we are smothering the other person with the intention - usually unconsciously - of making the

other person equal to ourselves, or even to overthrow him
so that we have a sense of our own even greater expansion
in the world. Another aspect is that basically we cannot
tolerate another person being different from ourselves and
having his own identity. If we do accept this, we become
aware of the chasm yawning between us and other people,
and this is very frightening. By making the other person
equal to ourselves, or by subjugating him, we thus not only
remove the threat of this chasm, but also the strange and
different aspect of that other person, and so have a sense of
connection.

This antisocial instinct in the field of the will is encoun-
tered everywhere in society. It is found between parents and
children, as well as between adults. It plays a role in sects
and in fascist groups, where the individuality of the members is sacrificed for the sake of the all-encompassing group
experience.

The effect of Ahriman can also be clearly recognized here
in the field of the will, as well as that of the Asurian forces.
Ahriman suppresses the individuality of the other person,
his views, feelings and behaviour, and punishes them, denies
them or mocks him. The Asurian forces are present particularly in those situations when the oppression or abuse of
another person goes so far that he is partly or wholly destroyed, and when this event gives feelings of pleasure or lust
when power or strength is derived from the victim.

Rudolf Steiner predicted that all these deep egoistic impulses will become much stronger than they are now. [62]
This is necessary because the human I and personality will
have to develop more powerfully if we, as people, are to
learn to become fully independent and bear the spirit alone
ourselves.

Self development

In the preceding chapters we saw that if we give our personal impulses free rein and do not work on them consciously, we become increasingly antisocial in our thoughts,
feelings and behaviour, and become increasingly locked up
inside ourselves. If we continue on this path, we will ultimately not only become utterly lonely and hardened as
individuals, but will also come to grief in conflict and in
wars with each other through the increasing power of the
counter-forces. If, on the other hand, we wish to follow the
path of development towards the spirit, we must consciously
work on ourselves and on forming real connections with
other human beings. What do we need for this?

In the first place, there is the goal of increasing self-
knowledge and honesty in our contact with other people. We
should recognize that our everyday personality always has
the tendency to use other people for its own feeling-experi-
ences. We should recognize the tendency of always putting
ourselves between the other person and our perception of
her or him, and see that we relate everything that is said to
ourselves. It is only with this self-knowledge that we will be
able to achieve a conscious approach in our encounters with
other people.

Then we can start to consciously practise using the
polarity between the social and the antisocial impulse. For
one person, this may mean that he will try not to lose
himself in the contact with other people, but tries to maintain this inner strength while opening up to other people.
For another person, whose nature tends more towards an
antisocial approach, the emphasis is rather on breaking

through his own isolation, and on becoming receptive towards other people.

In fact, every meeting with another person requires a consciousness of what should happen in this contact. We should ask ourselves: what is best here? Does the situation require me to be subjective, so that I step into my own experiences and the other person can get to know me, or is it actually better that the other person expresses himself and that I should relate to that objectively to make it possible? Should this be a one-way process, or should there be constant activity to and fro?

Thus, what is needed is that we should develop a feeling for that which the conversation or the meeting wants. In this way we will achieve the correct structure and tone for the conversation. If we relate to other people in this sort of conscious way, we will become aware that increasingly we will be able to successfully break through the resistances and forces of antipathy and sympathy in ourselves, so that we can open up to other people. On the other hand, by training our capacity to think clearly and our consciousness, we will develop the strength not to lose ourselves in the contact.

Thus, if we recognize our tendency to dominate others and use them for our own purposes in the field of the *will*, we can learn to restrain this tendency. This means that we create a space in which the other person can freely and unreservedly express himself and be himself.

We will be able to make increasingly good use of our *feelings,* if we recognise the need for us to experience ourselves, so that it becomes possible to handle this tendency and to learn to empathize with others in a free and objective way, and to be touched and moved by what the other person says.

Finally, we can also practise a different approach to *thinking.* This means consciously giving the other person the freedom and space to express his ideas, views and experiences, to share these inwardly, to help to formulate them and to try and understand them with our own thoughts.

If we live in other people in this selfless way, trying to experience and feel and think with them, and if we try to clarify and explain the situation by asking questions and looking for insights, we will gradually start to understand more and more about the other person. Through his words we will hear what he wishes to express and bring into his consciousness from the depths of his soul. By carefully feeling for and seeking answers to questions together in this way, and by 'sleeping into' in each other's experiences and then becoming conscious of them, we will achieve an ever deeper objective insight into the situation or the question. Finally we will reach the level of the spirit, where the truth, the essence of all experiences and perceptions, is expressed.

Therefore the important thing is, by means of empathizing and thinking with other people, to listen in such a way that a deeper insight can be achieved. In his book, *How to Know Higher Worlds,* Rudolf Steiner describes how the 'pupil' can develop the capacity to hear the essential elements in the words of another person on his path to inner development. I will quote a few extracts from this book because he indicates exactly what is important in this listening activity.

'For his inner development, the way in which a pupil *listens* to other people when they are speaking is extremely important. He should cultivate the habit of doing this in such a way that his own inner self remains completely *silent.* When one person expresses a view and another person is listening, there is usually a feeling of agreement or rejection in the latter. Many people will immediately feel the need to express their agreement, and more particularly, their rejection. A pupil should completely silence such disagreement or rejection. This does not mean that he suddenly has to change his lifestyle, constantly trying to achieve this deep inner silence. He should start by consciously choosing to practise this in particular circumstances. Very gradually, this new way of listening will automatically become habitual. It is not a matter merely of silencing only his intellectual views, but also every feeling of displeasure and rejection, as well as feelings of approval. In particular, the pupil should always carefully ensure that these feelings, even if they are not present on the surface, do not remain hidden in the inner depths of his soul. For example, he should listen to the views of people who are far below him in another respect, and then suppress *all* feelings of superiority or of knowing better (...) In this way the pupil will learn to listen to the words of another person in a completely *selfless* way, totally switching off his own personality, his own views and feelings. Anyone who practises listening in this way without any criticism, even to a view diametrically opposed to his own, or when he is confronted by the "most senseless" ideas, will slowly learn to fuse together with the essential aspect of the person, and to be taken up in that person. Then he will listen through the words into the other person's soul.'

Steiner says that by practising listening in this way,

'(...) a new sense of hearing comes to life in the soul. The soul becomes capable of hearing "words" from the spiritual world that are not expressed in outer tones and cannot be heard by physical ears. Perception of the "inner word" awakens. Truths are gradually revealed to us out of the spiritual world. We hear ourselves spoken to spiritually. All higher truths are attained only through such inward prompting.' [63]

However, for clarity's sake, he adds that the higher spiritual beings (which also include our own individual spiritual beings) speak only when someone is listening selflessly. As long as the listener still responds to what can be heard with a particular view or feeling, the beings of the spiritual world remain silent. [63]

As I described above, this inner speaking occurs when we raise our experiences to the level of the spirit, which then expresses the essences and truths hidden in it in our soul.

In the same book, Steiner wrote about the way in which we can develop our ability to *answer:*

'If someone says something to me that I must respond to, I must make an effort to pay more attention to the other person's beliefs, feelings and even prejudices than to anything I myself might add to the conversation at that moment. In other words, if one is on an occult path one must dedicate oneself conscientiously to schooling an impeccable sense of tact or delicacy. We must learn to gauge the significance for another person of having his or her opinion contradicted by ours. This does not mean that we should hold back our opinions. There is no question of that. But we should listen to the other person as carefully as possible and formulate our response on the basis of what we have heard.'

One particular idea can serve to point the direction in this respect:

'It does not matter if what I think differs from what the other person thinks. What matters is that, as a result of what I can contribute to the conversation, the other discovers what is right out of themselves.' [64]

Paths to Christ

The social path to Christ

The fact that we, as people who are naturally so involved with ourselves in an antisocial, selfish way, can nevertheless have contact with other people, is due to the Christ-impulse which lives within us. This gives us the possibility to build a bridge to the other person, and reach his or her inner spirit self in such a way that a completely new connection is formed both with the other and with our own inner spirit self.

Where does Christ's activity start in this social contact? It actually starts where it lives: in our own soul, in our own heart, and in that which emerges from that: our words. St. Paul wrote to the Romans: 'The word is nigh thee, even in thy mouth, and in thy heart.' [65] Rudolf Steiner also pointed out that the Christ impulse must be taken in with the forces of the heart if it is to become active in us. 'It is not the forces of the intellect, but the deepest forces of the soul and the heart which must take in the Christ impulse; and when it is taken in, it does not work in an individual human sense, but in a general human way.' [66] Thus he is saying that if we try to understand Christ only with the intellect, nothing happens, because he cannot act in this. However, he can come to life in our feelings and in our hearts. If we approach another person on the basis of the forces in the heart, the force of Christ himself works in this approach. However, this will not work only on the person at which it is aimed, but at the same time on the whole of humanity.

This means that the renewing force of Christ works in every sincere experience of another person's joy or pain, which comes to us from that other person, in every gesture of warmth we make to another person, and in every kind word we speak to another person. This force then not only benefits that person as a result of the gesture of interest or love, but also all people on earth. What we do to another person has direct consequences for the influence of Christ in the world, both in a positive and in a negative sense. 'Inasmuch as ye have done *unto one of the least of these my brethren, ye have done* unto me.' [67] This applies both in the material field and in the field of the spirit and the soul. According to Rudolf Steiner, in an age when the consciousness soul is developing, this sentence can be followed by another sentence: 'What ye have understood of the least of my brethren, ye have understood of me.' [68] This understanding, this approach in consciousness, is the precondition for social activity in our time.

This means that the more we do for another person, and understand about him, the stronger Christ can work between us on earth. Obviously the depth of this experience of this task is difficult to grasp immediately. Steiner wrote: 'This idea must be completely transformed into feeling, and only then can the truth of it be fully understood. What is revealed then makes all ideas and representations which divide people from each other disappear, and something common to all humanity surrounds the earth like an aura.' This is what happens when we seek Christ in the person facing us. [69]

These are the dimensions which apply when we talk about forces emanating from us, when Christ works through our heart, our words and our actions. What is important is not the particular faith we have, or the names we give to the divine element. The force of Christ lives in all men on earth, and it is active whenever the forces of the heart flow between people, whether they are Muslims, Jews, Buddhists, Christians or atheists.

This is why Rudolf Steiner called an interest in other people, the warm involvement in another person, the 'golden impulse of social life.' [70] This golden impulse of interest in other people, in their life, their circumstances, what moves them and the questions that they have – in other words, in everything that makes them the person they are – leads to an understanding of the being of that person. This understanding ensures that we will relate to her or him in the right way. A true interest in other people and in the things around us is, at the same time, the key to moral behaviour. It is clear that the heart of social life beats in the interest that one person feels for the other.

What helps a child, but also an adult, to progress in life? Anyone who has ever experienced that someone else truly 'saw' him and related to him with interest, knows the effect that this has had. Every adult will remember the one teacher who took a special interest in him at school. This made it possible to achieve things which were not possible with other teachers. For many people such stimulating experiences are a source of strength which later helped them to cope with difficult situations.

An interest is more than a sense of empathy. The feeling should be accompanied by an insight into the other person's situation and an understanding of the specific task that the person faces as a result of that situation. Only then will empathy have the desired effect.

This applies very clearly in the case of compassion. Compassion on its own may be forced upon one, or may be slightly insulting. Some people are particularly aware of themselves when they feel pity for someone else, or are reliving an earlier situation of their own in this feeling. There are also people who express their own need to take others under their wing in their feelings of pity. That is why there are many suffering people who do not want pity. However, they do want other people to take the trouble to understand them and their situation. Empathy or compassion which results from understanding does not have an oppressive or patronizing element, but has a liberating effect. Compassion which is the result of an insight into a situation is a liberating force and gives strength so that the situation can be more easily borne. The person who is suffering will feel this liberation, as well as a sense of real love: love which sees, knows, understands and gives strength. In this selfless, objective, liberating and yet understanding love, it is Christ himself who works; this can be *experienced* by anyone who is open to it.

When we wish to express the force of Christ with our heart, the real issue is whether we are able to develop an inner attitude towards other people which can be described as an attitude of benevolence. This is an attitude in which goodwill, good intentions to other people and the readiness to receive the other person's response with an open, mild acceptance are present. However, we do not naturally have such an open, attitude of benevolence. It develops only when we have gone through many painful and disappointing experiences, and when we have done a great deal of work on ourselves. In other words, when we have followed a path which has taught us to know and accept the strengths and weaknesses of other people, as well as our own strengths and weaknesses.

It is only then that we will be able to empathize with people in such a way that we can experience what they are experiencing as though it is happening to us. It becomes possible for us to forget ourselves out of inner strength, and to use the forces of our thoughts, feelings and our will to help other people to develop.

If we approach other people and their responses to us in this sort of benevolent manner, and if we allow these to live freely in the warm space of our hearts including their imperfections, we are acting in the sense of the Christ impulse.

Christ came down to earth and went through the crucifixion, death and resurrection on Golgotha as a divine being. In this way he connected with the inner aspect of the earth, mankind and each single human being. It is only through this divine act that human evolution is able to continue.

The above shows us even more clearly that in the declining world of the Father, Christ can only resurrect the warmth and light of the spirit if each of us personally learns to relate to other people in the right way. We can see that every gesture and every word which we utter to another person is of universal significance and determines the question whether Christ will be able to build the new and everlasting world of the spirit in our transient world.

If we listen, speak and act with other people in such a way that Christ can work through us in our interest, love and understanding, we will contribute to this new world. When we ignore our fellow man, show no love or interest in him, we contribute to the further destruction of the old world by the counterforces. Parts of this world in which since Golgotha the Christ-forces live, then become possessed.[71] It is not for nothing that it is often said that Christ was first crucified on Golgotha, but that he is being crucified again and again by our own thoughts and actions.

This is why the whole future of mankind can always be brought back to the question of our own personal development. The new world starts in ourselves. When we realize this, we will get to the point where we become really concerned, when we do not feel that our interest and involvement in other human beings becomes stronger every day.

Impotence and resurrection

In our time there are many paths leading to Christ and to an encounter with him in our own souls. One of these is the path of the crisis. We experience more and more crises in our personal life. They bring a sense of being stuck, of not being able to go on, of standing on the edge of an abyss. Unconsciously, we are experiencing the withdrawal of the ancient, supportive and protective forces of the sphere of the Father. If, at the same time, the new forces of the spirit working within are still insufficiently present in our inner selves, there is a void in the soul, a void which can be felt as an abyss in certain circumstances. Where does this experience come from?

Our personality, our normal self, is based in the first instance in the physical body. Our thoughts are connected with the nerves and sensory system, our emotions with the rhythmic processes of the lungs and the heart, while the will has a connection with the metabolism and the limbs. These close links between physical processes and soul processes mean that changes in one area have repercussions for the other. For example, the withdrawal of the forces of the Father from the physical body has great consequences for the development of our soul and personality. One of these consequences is that the structures which hold our personality together become weaker. This can go so far that at a certain point the personality falls apart. How is this possible?

We saw that our personality consists of two separate parts. One part, which is still very small, already contains some of the spiritual substance and strength of our higher being, our spirit self, as a result of the work we have done on ourselves.

This is not yet the case in the other part of the personality, which is by far the larger. This still consists predominantly of a coarse soul substance of undigested impressions and experiences, and other unconscious aspects of the soul.

In the part of our personality which already contains an aspect of the spiritual being, spiritual substance which is indestructible and eternal, is already present. Therefore that part of our personality cannot fall apart, and the counter-forces cannot grasp it. However, the other part of the personality, which has its basis still entirely in the physical body is extremely vulnerable. In times when we have many psychological shocks to deal with, it can simply fall apart sooner or later. This may happen when a person, or an animal we love, dies, when we go through a divorce or another traumatic experience, when we feel deeply hurt or humiliated, and so on. It can also happen during the transitional stages of life, for example, during puberty or in the mid-life crisis.

People whose personality has partly fallen apart feel that they are made up of several different inner pieces, and that there is a dark, yawning abyss surrounding them, which imprisons them in a static, motionless state. This condition engenders fear, and people in this situation feel an existential fear of losing themselves, and despair, because they do not know what is happening to them, and how they will ever get out of this state.

Often they hear voices or see visions which may make them even more afraid. Some voices and images may remove them from the situation and take them into inner worlds where they have fantastic experiences, so that they may have a sense of being specially chosen. When this illusion passes, they fall back into even greater paralysis and a deeper void. Another sort of voice tells them in a hateful, cynical or mocking tone that they should not imagine they will ever be able to leave this state behind. These voices whisper that they are absolutely worthless as human beings, that they will never manage anything, and that life has absolutely no meaning or significance. These voices and images come from the counter-forces which rise up from the depths of the soul in these turbulent times, and spread their influence in people. In the elevated feelings and illusions of the first sort we recognize the hand of Lucifer. The oppressive influences of the second sort are characteristic of the work of Ahriman. More and more people are having these sorts of experiences nowadays.

If we are able to survive the inner crisis, in other words, if we have the courage and strength to pass through the experience of chaos, fear and despair, again and again, thus also overcoming the confrontation with the counter-forces, something eventually happens. Gradually, something rises up from deep inside us, which provides inner support and inner strength. This inner strength comes from our higher, spirit self. Each time we pass through the abyss, it is born in us a little more. This is why we emerge slightly stronger from all our painful experiences.

As a result of this process of passing through the abyss, we become aware that there are two sorts of forces in us. One sort takes us to a particular end point in ourselves. The other leads us on.

The first sort makes us experience a process of death in the soul. In this situation we feel that we cannot go on, that everything in us is being extinguished, and that at this point we might die. Many people who are in this sort of situation literally describe it in these terms. It is an experience that is accompanied by a deep feeling of inner darkness in which we feel abandoned by God and everyone. Our will is paralysed, and we experience a profound sense of impotence.

This feeling is produced by an unconscious knowledge that we are no longer able to find the path to the divine world with our ordinary self, which is based on our mortal, physical body. We realize that actually everything ends there. This experience of death and feeling of impotence expresses a profound reality: it indicates how sick the mortal part of our soul and our I and personality really are. This sickness

is related to what was traditionally called 'the Fall', the state
which arose because the counter-forces gained a hold,
during the course of evolution, over our physical body, and
thence over our soul and our I. The result is that with this
part of ourselves, we can no longer experience ourselves as
fundamentally divine beings. That is why so many people
nowadays deny the existence of God and the spiritual world.

When we have really lived through this feeling of impotence, a fundamental change happens. We become aware
that in the middle of this process of death, this petrified
impotence, a force is slowly growing from inside, giving us
strength and support. It is as though we are being reborn,
and a strength is aroused in us which enables us to lift our
head, look around us with new eyes, and have the courage
to take new steps.

When we experience both these feelings consciously in our
soul – the sense of impotence, the inability to go on, the
sickness, on the one hand, and the force which conquers
this impotence and heals the sickness, on the other hand, we
have found the reality of Christ in ourselves. Rudolf Steiner
wrote:

'(...) When we experience a feeling of impotence and the
recovery from this impotence, we have the good fortune
of discovering a true relationship with Jesus Christ (...)
Seek in yourself and you shall find impotence. Seek, and
you shall find, after you have found the impotence, the
deliverance from this impotence, the resurrection of the
soul to the spirit.' [72]

Experiences such as these make us aware that Christ lives in
our own soul since Golgotha. He lives in that part of us
which is vulnerable, where there is the abyss, the darkness,
the abandonment by God, inner death. Living in our soul he
experiences everything we experience. He knows what we
think, what we feel, what goes through us, what we want,
and what we need. He also consoles us when we are troubled,
protects us and gives us new vital strength.

We are unaware, or hardly aware of any of this. It is as though there is a thin wall between him and us which prevents us from directly experiencing who he is and what he is doing. However, there are occasional times when the wall becomes transparent for a moment and we suddenly become aware of his being. Increasing numbers of people are experiencing this nowadays. However, we will be able to experience the forces emanating from Christ much more directly if we can open up inwardly and consciously seek to make contact with him. In this way, the wall separating us from him becomes thinner. On the other side, Christ is also approaching us. Thus we will be able to perceive him more clearly in the future, and we will know from our own experience that he lives and is with us.

The personal path to Christ

We can only start to understand who Christ is, how he works in us, and the mystery of Golgotha when we have lived through the experience of impotence and the resurrection following upon this. Then we will find increasing certainty that the force of inner spiritual resurrection is the result of Christ's act on Golgotha. This experience is, as it were, the archetype of the path by which we can find Christ.

How can we join Christ in a personal and increasingly conscious way? In the first place, we can do this by submitting our needs to him, and asking him questions about all sorts of problems of life. This means that we can share with him our burdens and worries, our fears and shortcomings, our feelings of inadequacy and guilt. In addition, we can then freely ask for insights and for advice, strength and support for all sorts of things which affect our lives. If we do this correctly, in other words, not in an intellectual or abstract way, but in such a way that we have an inner experience of these worries and questions, we can be certain that Christ will answer them. However, we should not expect that we will immediately hear or see him. Christ himself chooses the way in which he gives answers, but he will always answer with a stream of strength, a strengthening of our soul and new impulses for our lives.

In the words of Rudolf Steiner: 'Christ is not only a leader of human beings, he is also a brother of human beings who wishes to be consulted, who particularly wishes to be consulted in the times to come about all the specific aspects of life.' Then it may happen that:

'(...) the human being sees Christ by his side as a loving companion, and receives not only consolation and strength from the Christ being, but also a clarification about what has to happen.' If our questions are asked in a sufficiently serious way, we can be sure that Christ will answer them. 'He will answer, he will truly give an answer, and anyone who asks for Christ's advice in the twilight of the spirit which lives in the depths of our times will receive a rich source of strength and support and a wealth of impulses for his soul.'

Secondly, we can come closer to Christ by trying to experience something of his essence in ourselves. We can do this, for example, by reading the Bible or other books about the life and work of Christ, and by reflecting on and living through the contents of these books. We also join him when we pray to him, when we meditate and immerse ourselves in his being during moments of inner peace and quiet, so opening up to him. And we open up to his supportive strength when we say the prayer 'Our Father' together with him, the prayer which Christ himself gave to mankind.[73] 'Our Father' is a prayer which strengthens the forces of light in the world, and therefore also gives us strength in times of need.

Above all, we join Christ when we not only try to experience him, but also consciously take him into our will, and endeavour to allow his divine healing powers to work on earth through us. This 'path of the will' to Christ is obviously a tremendous task. It means that we have to change ourselves profoundly. It requires us to shape our thoughts, feelings, words and I in such a way that Christ can think, experience and speak through us. It means also that we must develop our actions and behaviour in such a way that the strength of Christ can flow through our will and actions.[74]

With the 'path of the will' to Christ, we have arrived at the point where the personal path to Christ turns into the social path. The fact that this is so is related to the essence of Christ himself. He at the same time lives in every single human being, and also between them, and therefore in humanity as a whole. As the divine 'I am', he is the divine I which is the fundamental basis of every person.[75] That is why every individual can become conscious of her- or himself and experience the true self, the spirit self, in the soul. However, because the I of humanity, Christ, lives in each of us and joins us together on the level of the invisible, we can always find the path to each other, even though we may be strangers to one another for some time.

The brotherhood of human beings

The essence of the personal path to Christ is that I place myself in his service, while retaining my own individual self, in the sense of the words of St. Paul: 'Not I, but Christ liveth in me.'[(76)] On this path, I personally endeavour to live not only for myself, but also to increase and strengthen my skills and consciousness in such a way that I am able to encompass and carry an increasingly large part of creation. Thus on this path to Christ, I acquire a sense of responsibility for everything that lives and is developing. Apart from other people, this also includes other creatures of nature, such as plants and animals, as well as the earth as a living organism.

On the social path to Christ the true aim is to develop and give such form and content to the contacts or encounters with other people that the strength of Christ can work between them and me in the sense: 'Where two or more are gathered in my name, there I am in the midst of them.' [77] On the social path to Christ, I try to put this sense of responsibility for all living things into practice also by my actions. If I do this in such a way that Christ can work through me, the living, divine spirit is awoken and raised up in the other person, in nature and in the animals and plants.

In this way we are able to actively participate in the transformation of the transient world of the Father into the eternal world of the Spirit of Christ. The earth and everything which lives on there are thus protected from destruction, and the future planetary stages of the earth and higher states of consciousness of man can be prepared in the mortal nature of the human being and the earth. It shows that we human beings are closely involved in this new creation. With our moral acts we lay the spiritual foundation for future lives and worlds. For the morality of today forms the germ of later external realities.[78] Christ assimilates the acts which we have performed with insight and with loving involvement, and from this forms the nature of the new earth, of the new developmental stage of our planet. Because it comes from Christ, this future nature will radiate love and morality everywhere, just as we encounter wisdom everywhere in the present nature of the earth.[79]

The basis of all these developments is that during the events on Golgotha, Christ not only united with humanity as a whole and with the earth, but also with each person individually. He lives in everything and is the same for all living creatures, and yet he is a 'personal matter' for each individual.[80] That is why we can feel personally involved with everything that lives, and gradually we will be able to take increasing responsibility for the larger whole of mankind and nature.

All around us we can see that people are undergoing a spiritual awakening in this field. As a result of the liberation of the inner spirit, the sense of responsibility for the surrounding natural world and for the needs of our fellow human beings on earth is constantly increasing. The activities of international organizations such as Greenpeace and Amnesty International confirm this. More and more people are following the personal and social path to Christ, even though they may not be aware of it. In them, there is a concern for the future of the earth and of nature, and for the free spiritual development of mankind. This non-exclusive concern reflects the Christian impulse.

This sense of responsibility for everything that lives could also be called a feeling of brotherhood for our fellow human beings. Brotherhood between human beings develops when we recognize in the other those things which also live in us, and that we therefore have in common. This sort of experience leads to a completely new sort of friendship between people, a friendship which not only has a starting point in the soul and in empathy with others, but, because we really come to know each other, also grows in the spirit. This produces a deep sense of mutual involvement and togetherness. We recognize how the spirit becomes more and more human in the other person and is gradually increasingly clearly expressed. This experience evokes a sense of wonder and awe. Awe, because we are aware of the difficult and painful path which must be followed before the inner being is born; wonder, respect and enthusiasm, because we experience how the spirit appears in the other person in an entirely new and individual way, revealing the divine element in a human being. The sense of brotherhood which is created in this way means that I start to feel responsible for the other person, for his or her welfare, development and existence.

The sense of brotherhood in relation to other people does not mean that we find each other's shortcomings and one-sidedness easy to deal with. At the level of the ordinary personality, those parts which have not yet been liberated inevitably cause dissent and strife. This is inherent to the present stage of our development. However, by showing our friction and collisions in the light of the path of development we are both following, we can always find a way out. It is a matter of insight - into ourselves, into the other person, and what has ensnared us both - but also a question of goodwill. We must be prepared and able to find the other person again and again, to conquer the problems and resistances and to talk about the things which have come between us. Then we will not resent the pain the other person has caused us, and we will be able to forgive each other.[81] By learning to relate to each other in this way, the sense of brotherly connection will become a constantly recurring experience.

However, the main thing on the path to brotherhood is the struggle to achieve insight and understanding. We must learn to step out of ourselves and try to understand the thoughts, the feelings and the experiences of the other person through the path of spiritual knowledge.

If I immerse myself in an unselfish way in that which moves the other, in what has happened in her or his life, in how she or he relates to all kinds of things in life, and lift these experiences up to the level of spiritual insight, I awaken the other person in the deepest level of her or his soul. And that is not all.

At the same time, this true image also leads me to a sense of connection with this other person and a sense of brotherhood. This happens because the Christ then works in me. When I strive to develop a true image of the other person in an unselfish, yet conscious and active way, it is Christ in me, in us, who can then connect us people who have become so separated from each other, in a new, free way. A way in which we both keep our independence as individuals.

The more we build true images of each other the more the spirit self awakens in the individuals and the more we human beings get connected again in new, free bonds of brotherhood.

As Steiner wrote, creating images of each other means that person A is no longer in one place, person B in another, and person C somewhere else again, separately and unrelated to each other, but that A and B come alive in C, A in C and B, and so on. The more we connect again in this conscious way, the greater the sense of brotherhood between human beings will become. Steiner wrote:

'We can only speak of brotherhood between men - which was initially merely an empty cliché - if we carry that other person in us as our self. If we form an image of that other person which is planted in our soul as a treasure, we carry part of him in our soul, just as we carry something of our physical brother in our blood. Instead of merely blood relationships, spiritual relationships should form the basis of social life in this concrete way. This is something which truly has to develop.' [82]

If we human beings become spiritual brothers, we also become brothers of Christ at the same time, for '(...) Christ wishes to recognize as his brother, the person who recognizes someone else as his brother.' [83] This interconnection between human beings which does not only comprise that which is good and pure, but also that which is imperfect and bad, allows us to form a direct relationship with Christ: 'By this shall all men know that ye are my disciples, if ye have love one to another.' [84]

Christ can work in our midst when we human beings are connected in a brotherly way. The fact that this is possible is based on a general spiritual law. People who share something together, such as an ideal, a study or a common task, and therefore interact with each other, create a spiritual body as a group which then becomes linked to a spiritual being. If the correct conditions are met, this being is Christ. Regardless of the question whether the members themselves have a connection with Christ, if the correct conditions are met, they are gathered in his name and then Christ is among them.

Rudolf Steiner formulated the spiritual law related to group formation in the following way: 'Unification means the possibility that a higher being expresses itself through the united members. This is a general principle of life. Five people who are together .... are not simply the sum of five, just as our body is not merely the sum of our five senses. That living together, that interconnectedness of human beings with each other, corresponds to the interconnectedness of the cells of the human body. A new, higher being is present among those five persons, and even amongst two or three.' [85]

We refer to this law when we use phrases such as 'family feeling', a club spirit or team spirit. These reveal an aspect of a spiritual reality which is expressed in a particular family or in the members of a particular group, a spirit which connects the members of the group together, and gives them something in common.

The spiritual force which connects a group together can take many different forms. It can be a giving force, giving the members strength, freedom and inspiration. But it can also take and remove strength and energy from them, and even work in a destructive way.

The quality of a spiritual being connecting to a group is determined by the moral quality of the people who come together, and the way in which they deal with each other. Anyone with experience of groups will be familiar with this phenomenon. If the members of a group are not interested in each other, if there is no mutual trust, if the 'conversation' is mainly 'silence', or consists of only expressing individual views and opinions, then the people concerned go home empty. They feel that they have not got any further, and even have a sense of loss. This experience is even stronger when in such a group there is also an atmosphere of distrust, criticism and condemnation, because people are unable to control their antipathetic feelings. In such groups, the antisocial element predominates, and then in a spiritual sense a 'hole' is formed in the middle which sucks away every contribution or attempt to contribute. Nothing can develop. Conversations never really start, and the people involved feel paralysed and separated from each other by an unbridgeable chasm. Afterwards, some may feel that inwardly they are broken into different pieces, or feel as though they are standing on the edge of an abyss. The meeting of the group and the group spirit has broken something inwardly. It may take quite a while before they are whole again and regain their former strength. Clearly it was not a spirit from the world of light that was present in this group, but a spirit from the domains where the counter-forces operate.

In fact, we ourselves determine by our behaviour and our way of dealing with each other which spiritual forces will connect with the groups of which we are a member. These groups of course also include our personal relationships with other individuals.

Traditionally, church communities have been the groups which made it possible for Christ to work on earth. The communal celebration of the Mass or service in the Protestant church created an opportunity for divine beings such as Christ to be present among those who were assembled. In our time, in which Christ is revealing himself more and more, this opportunity becomes increasingly possible in daily encounters with other human beings. That is what Rudolf Steiner meant when he said that in the future, '(...) every encounter between one human being and the other will be a religious act, a sacrament.' [86]

This is why we can consciously choose to form groups which are aimed at creating a place for Christ to work on earth, in addition to having a more obvious raison d'être.

Of course, such groups can be formed on all sorts of themes. They may be aimed at studying spiritual or religious subjects, and relating these to the members' own experiences. They may be groups in which people talk together about their lives, forming insights and supporting each other in their individual development. They may also be groups which are aimed at working in an innovative way at every level of society, for example in agriculture, health or education. Finally, they may also be groups in which the members rarely meet in a physical sense, though they support each other's inner development or work towards a higher goal with united strength. The thing which all these groups have in common is their unselfish endeavours to achieve a goal which transcends the personal interests.

When does Christ work in such a group of people? This happens when these people create the above-mentioned conditions for meeting and encounter. When those who meet together are aware of their own anti-social forces and can control these to a large extent, while they at the same time develop social skills that enable them to build the bridge to the other person to understand him or her, this results in an open and well-meaning atmosphere in which the group can become a group in the true sense. This attitude results in a lively and committed interaction between those who are present. An interaction in which the participants on the basis of each other's experiences, thoughts and feelings seek for new insights and new ways of dealing with things together. If this happens in such a way that every participant has the feeling that he or she is seen or heard by the others and is approached with understanding, then Christ is present. In the participants the working of his spirit flames up and so they become connected with their spirit self. They feel that they can be themselves, and have a sense of freedom. They notice that thinking and speaking become easy. The brotherly attitude and activities of the others around her or him loosens the tongue, creating a feeling of trust. This means that the Spirit inspires them and that truth can be found. Those who are present then gain insights into things which they did not understand or know before.

A good example of this spiritual effect can be seen in the dialogues which I had with the thirteen-year-old boy. The same process occurred in a striking, but all the more recognisable way in the group which was studying the social impulse of Anthroposophy. The difficulties and problems which the participants had struggled to overcome together, conquering their own antisocial impulses, and the efforts to get through to the other and keep her or him involved in the process, resulted in the spirit of Christ becoming active in the group. The sparks of inspiration not only provided insights into their questions, through knowledge and direct experience, but also connected them with their inner spiritual being and therefore in a new way also with each other.

Experiences such as these, which were first experienced by the disciples at Pentecost - though of course in a much more fundamental way - will become common among humans. Two thousand years ago it was still an experience reserved for a chosen group, but nowadays it is within reach of every human being because of the new way in which Christ works. The experiences I described before give only a very faint indication of what we will experience now that the working of Christ becomes stronger every day. If we create the correct conditions, he will appear in our midst and can be perceived even in a visible form wherever and whenever we meet in his name. This is the great time we are moving towards.

When this event happens we will then experience a source of strength and inspiration working in our midst, which will feed us all. This inspiration will work in such a way that it will give us insights into questions, problems and circumstances that we meet in life. We will receive consolation and encouragement, enabling us to face the tasks of life with renewed energy. We will gain inner strength and spiritual nourishment which will affect the organs of our physical body through our soul, filling them with new spiritual energy. However, this spiritual benefit will not be restricted to this single group. The divine substance which is created here will also be used by Christ to work in other fields on the progress of the human evolution.

In this context there is another very important point. At meetings where we come together in a brotherly way, we not only enable Christ to be present, but we also create connections with Michael, the time spirit, and his angels. When Christ is working amongst us a bridge is built from us to the world of the spirit. This is a connecting channel through which the higher angel beings of light and progress can descend to earth, led by Michael, to work on the continued development of humanity, together with Christ. Michael is then able to fight the forces of evil on earth, and to support the human beings in their struggle.

Rudolf Steiner wrote: 'Thus human connections are the secret place where high spiritual beings descend to work through individual people, just as the spirit works through our limbs.' [87] He added elsewhere: 'People who connect with other people, and who use their strength for all, are those who lay the foundations for the correct development for the future.' [88]

At the moment we are still living in an era in which the consciousness soul is being developed. This is the so-called fifth cultural epoch which stretches from the end of the Middle Ages to halfway through the fourth millennium. At the same time we are already sowing the seeds for the next cultural period, which has been called the 'social age'. In the Revelation of St. John, this is called the community of Philadelphia, the community of brotherly love. In a lecture in 1908, Rudolf Steiner said of this period: '(...) this sixth cultural age will be an extremely important one because it will bring peace and brotherhood through communal wisdom.' In the future, wisdom will be a common attribute to a much greater extent than it is now, because people will constantly raise up their experiences to a spiritual level. They will discover that the ultimate truth can be found in one's own soul, but also that this truth is the same for all people, just as mathematical truths are now. This experience will result in a feeling of peace and brotherliness, 'because the higher self will in its elementary form as the spirit self or *manas* for the first time enter not only in a few chosen people, but in that part of humanity which goes through a normal development. A connection will be formed between the I of the human being as he has gradually developed, and the higher self.' [90]

When we unite as human beings to achieve this future, we are joining all those who have undertaken this task throughout the centuries of Christianity. There were many different movements and groups who did this, from the Manichaeans and Celtic monks to the Rosicrucians and the Knights Templar. We must continue the work started by these groups in a contemporary way.

If we take up the personal and social tasks that lie ahead, there will be a tremendous release of spiritual strength in our hearts and souls. Through this a society of human beings will be established on earth in which the divine Sophia, the Holy Spirit sent by Christ, will become alive and active. A society of individuals bound in a brotherly way and who through the bright light of their thoughts and the warmth and strength of their hearts enable the divine Spirit to illuminate, to warm and to guide the progress of humanity.

We are all called upon to contribute to this future, as well as we can.

Notes

1. Hans Stolp, *Dichterbij dan ooit*, Uitgeverij Ten Have, Baarn 1989.

2. For the literature on the Trinity, see Hans-Werner Schroeder, *Drieëenheid en drievuldigheid, Het geheim van de triniteit*, Zeist, 1994 Oskar Kürten, *Der Sohnesgott, der Logos und die Trinität*, Basle 1983; Rudolf Steiner, *Das Geheimnis der Trinität*, Rudolf Steiner Gesamtausgabe (GA), no. 214, Dornach 1980.

3. See St. Paul's First Letter to the Corinthians 8 : 6.

4. St. John 1 : 1-3. See also 'Christus ist auferstanden', interview with Hans-Werner Schroeder in *Flensburger Hefte* 39, 1992.

5. Jean Gebser, *Ursprung und Gegenwart*, Gesamtausgabe parts II and III, Schaffhausen 1978.

6. Rudolf Steiner, *De geestelijke leiding van mens en mensheid*, Zeist 1993. *The Spiritual Guidance of Man*, ed Henry B. Monger, Anthroposophic Press, New York, 1983

7. See Rudolf Steiner, *Das Ereignis der Christus-Erscheinung in der Ätherischen Welt*, Rudolf Steiner Gesamtausgabe (GA), no. 118, Dornach 1984, lecture of 15 May 1910, *The Reappearance of Christ in the Etheric World*, Introduction by René Querido, Anthroposophic Press, New York, 1983, and *Das Geheimnis der Trinität*, Rudolf Steiner Gesamtausgabe (GA), no. 214, Dornach 1980, lecture of 30 July 1992. *The Mystery of the Trinity*, tr. George Adams, Rudolf Steiner Press, London, 1947.

8. Emil Bock, *De jaarfeesten als kringloop door het jaar,* Zeist 1990, the chapters 'Pinksteren, het feest der toekomst' and 'Heilige Geest - Helende Geest'.

9. Revelations 21 : 5.

10. See note 7, *The Reappearance of Christ in the Etheric World,* ibid, and note 8. Moreover,in addition to the spirit self, Steiner distinguishes two other essential spiritual aspects, the 'spirit life' and 'spirit body' or 'spirit man', which will develop at a later stage in evolution; see, inter alia, *Rudolf Steiner Theosophy,* Anthroposophic Press, New York, 1994.

11. See Rudolf Steiner, *How to Know Higher Worlds,* Anthroposophic Press, New York, 1995, *Wege und Ziele des geistigen Menschen,* GA 125, Dornach 1992, lecture 4 June 1910; *Die okkulten Grundlagen der Bhagavad Gita,* GA 146, Dornach 1992, lecture 30 May 1913 or *The Occult Significance of the Bhagaved Gita,* Anthroposophic Press, New York, 1968.

12. Rudolf Steiner, *Lectures on the Gospel According to St. John,* lectures of 19 and 26 May 1908.

13. Rudolf Steiner, *A Philosophy of Freedom, Intuitive Thinking as a Spiritual Path,* Anthroposophic Press, New York, 1995, chapters II and V.

14. *Das Hereinwirken geistiger Wesenheiten in den Menschen,* GA 102, Dornach 1984, lecture of 24 March 1908.

15. See Sergej O. Prokofieff, *The Circle of the Year as a Path of Initiation,* chapter V, Temple Lodge, London, 1995 and Stuttgart 1989, chapter V, and *The Occult Significance of Forgiveness,* chapter VI, V, Temple Lodge, London, 1993.

16. See Dieter Brüll, *De sociale impuls van de antroposofie,* Zeist 1985, introduction.

17. See Rudolf Steiner, *Metamorphoses of the Soul,* vols 1 and 2, Rudolf Steiner Press, London, lecture of 25 November 1909.

18. See, i.a., Rudolf Steiner, *From Jesus to Christ,* Rudolf Steiner Press, London, 1973, lectures of 9 and 10 October 1911, and Hans-Werner Schroeder, *De mens en het kwaad,* Zeist 1987, chapter 5.

19. See note 18, Schroeder.

20. Rudolf Steiner, *Cosmosophy,* Vol I, Anthroposophic Press, New York, 1985, GA 207, Dornach 1990, lectures of 23 and 24 September 1921.

21. Rudolf Steiner, *The Deed of Christ and the Opposing Spiritual Powers,* Steiner Book Centre Inc., Vancouver, 1976, GA 107, Dornach 1988, lecture of 22 March 1909.

22. Rudolf Steiner, *The Fall of the Spirits of Darkness,* Rudolf Steiner Press, Bristol, 1993, GA 177, Dornach 1985, lecture of 7 October 1917.

23. See Rudolf Steiner, *From Jesus to Christ,* op.cit., lecture of 13 October 1911, and *Erfahrungen des Übersinnlichen. Die Wege der Seele zu Christus,* GA143, lecture of 16 April 1912.

24. St. Matthew 28 : 20.

25. See, in particular, Rudolf Steiner, *The Reappearance of Christ in the Etheric World,* op.cit.

26. Matthew 24 : 30, Revelations 1 : 7.

27. See note 25.

28. *The Reappearance of Christ in the Etheric World,* op.cit., lecture of 25 January 1910.

29. *The Reappearance of Christ in the Etheric World,* op.cit., lecture of 27 January 1910.

30. *Esoteric Christianity and the Mission of Christian Rosenkreutz,* Rudolf Steiner Press, London, 1984, GA 130, Dornach 1987, lecture of 1 October 1911.

31. See note 30.

32. *Building Stones for an Understanding of the Mystery ofGolgatha,* Rudolf Steiner Press, London, lecture of 6 February 1917.

33. Hans Stolp, *Kijk, maar kijk met verwondering,* Ten Have Baarn 1990.

34. Rudolf Steiner, *Occult Science,* London, 1969, chapter II.

35. Rudolf Steiner, *How to Know Higher Worlds,* Anthroposophic Press, New York, 1995.

36. *Die Mystik im Aufgange des neuzeitlichen Geisteslebens und ihr Verhältnis zur modernen Weltanschauung,* GA 7, Dornach 1987, introduction.

37. See Rudolf Steiner, *Metamorphoses of the Soul,* op.cit., lecture of 5 December 1909.

37a M. Lefébre OP, Dr H. Schauder, *Conversations on Counselling,* T & T Clark, Edinburgh, 1990

38. See *Metamorphoses of the Soul,* op. cit. lecture of 14 March 1910.

39. See note 34.

40. *Theosophy,* Chapter II, Anthroposophic Press, New York, 1994.

41. See note 14. Also see Rudolf Steiner, *Apocalypse of St. John,* Rudolf Steiner Press, London, 1977, lecture of 27 December 1917; lecture of 30 June 1908. Also see *Der Jahreskreislauf als Einweihungsweg zum Erleben der Christuswesenheit,* Stuttgart 1989, chapters IX-1, XI-5 and especially 'Anmerkungen und Ergänzungen', no. 74, p. 425.

42. Rudolf Steiner, *Awakening to Community,* Anthroposophic Press, New York, 1974, GA 257, lectures of 27 February and 13 March 1923.

43. Rudolf Steiner, *Anthroposophical Leading Thoughts,* Rudolf Steiner Press, London, 1973, the 'Letter to the Members' of 23 March 1924.

44. See note 42.

45. See Rudolf Steiner, *Practical Training in Thinking,* Anthroposophic Press, New York, 1977.

46. See note 36.

47 Rudolf Steiner, *How to Know Higher Worlds,* Anthroposophic Press, New York, 1995.

47a Rudolf Steiner, *The Christian Mystery of the Resurrection and the Pre-Christian Mysteries,* Zeist 1985, p. 36 et seq.

48. Romans 8 : 119-23.

49. *Anthroposophical Leading Thoughts,* 19 and 25 October 1924.

50. See Rudolf Steiner, *The Riddles of Philosophy,* Anthroposophic Press, New York, 1973.

51. *The Mystery of the Trinity,* Rudolf Steiner Press, London, 1947, lecture of 27 August 1922.

52. See *Anthroposophical Leading Thoughts,* 19 October 1924.

53. See *Anthroposophical Leading Thoughts,,* 25 October 1924.

54. See note 51.

55. *The Challenge of the Times,* Anthroposophic Press, New York, n.d., GA 186, Dornach 1990, lecture of 29 November 1918.

56. *The Challenge of the Times,* Anthroposophic Press, New York, n.d., lectures of 6 and 12 December 1918 (the quotation is from the latter). On the subject of the 'social basic phenomenon', also see Dieter Brüll, *De sociale impuls van de antroposofie,* Zeist 1985; Friedrich Benesch, *Gemeenschapzin en individualisme,* Zeist 1988; Harry Salman, *Het beeld van de ander,* Leiden 1992.

57. See Rudolf Steiner, *Spiritual Scientific Knowledge and Social Understanding,* Typescript Z431.

58. See note 57.

59. *The Challenge of the Times,* 6 December 1918, Anthroposophic Press, New York, n.d.

60. See note 59.

61. *Social and Anti-Social Forces in the Human Being,* 12 December, Mercury Press, Spring Valley, 1982

62. See note 61.

63. *How to Know Higher Worlds,* op.cit., p. 48.

64. *How to Know Higher Worlds,* op.cit., p. 90-91.

65. Romans 10 : 8.

66. Rudolf Steiner, *Karmic Relationships,* Vol VI, Rudolf Steiner Press, London, 1989.,GA 240, Dornach 1977, lecture of 25 January 1924.

67. Matthew 25 : 40.

68. Rudolf Steiner, *Die soziale Frage als Bewusstseinfrage,* GA 189, Dornach 1980, lecture of 26 February 1919.

69. Rudolf Steiner, *Karma of Vocation in Connection with the Life of Goethe,* Anthroposophic Press, New York, 1995, lecture of 27 November 1916.

70. Rudolf Steiner, *Christ and the Human Soul,* Rudolf Steiner Press, London, 1972, lecture of 30 May 1912.

71. See note 70.

72. Rudolf Steiner, *Der Tod als Lebenswandlung,* GA 182, Dornach 1986, lecture of 16 October 1918.

73. Matthew 6 and Luke 11.

74. See Rudolf Steiner, *Geistige Zusammenhänge in der Gestaltung des menschlichen Organismus,* GA 218, Dornach 1992, lecture of 18 November 1922.

75. See Rudolf Steiner, *Occult Science - an Outline,* Anthroposophic Press, New York, 1962, chapter IV, and *Das esoterische Christentum und die geistige Führung der Menschheit,* GA 130, Dornach 1987, lecture of 9 January 1912.

76. Letters to the Galatians, 2 : 20.

77. Matthew 18 : 20.

78. See, i.a., Rudolf Steiner, *Karma of Vocation,* op.cit.

79. See, i.a., Rudolf Steiner, *Occult Science,* op.cit., chapter VI, and *The Gospel of St. John,* Anthroposophic Press, New York, 1962, lecture of 20 May 1908.

80. Rudolf Steiner, *The Mission of the Archangel Michael,* Anthroposophic Press, New York, 1961, lecture of 14 December 1919.

81. See Sergei O. Prokofieff, *The Occult Significance of Forgiveness,* op.cit.

82. *The Challenge of the Times,* 7 December 1918, op.cit.

83. Rudolf Steiner, *Preparing for the Sixth Epoch,* Anthroposophic Press, New York, 1976, lecture of 15 June 1915.

84. John, 13 : 35.

85. Rudolf Steiner, *Brotherhood and the Struggle for Existence,* Mercury Press, Spring Valley, 1980, lecture of 23 November 1905. Also see *Natuurwezens,* Zeist 1993, lectures of 1 and 7 June 1908.

86. Rudolf Steiner, *The Work of the Angels in Man's Astral Body,* Rudolf Steiner Press, London, 1972.

87. See note 85.

88. Rudolf Steiner, *Zur Geschichte und aus den Inhalten der erkenntniskultischen Abteilung der Esoterischen Schule von 1904 bis 1914,* GA 265, Dornach 1987, p. 125.

89. Revelations 3 : 7.

90. Rudolf Steiner, *The Gospel of St. John,* op.cit.

A note from the publisher

For more than a quarter of a century, **Temple Lodge Publishing** has made available new thought, ideas and research in the field of spiritual science.

Anthroposophy, as founded by Rudolf Steiner (1861-1925), is commonly known today through its practical applications, principally in education (Steiner-Waldorf schools) and agriculture (biodynamic food and wine). But behind this outer activity stands the core discipline of spiritual science, which continues to be developed and updated. True science can never be static and anthroposophy is living knowledge.

Our list features some of the best contemporary spiritual-scientific work available today, as well as introductory titles. So, visit us online at **www.templelodge.com** and join our emailing list for news on new titles.

If you feel like supporting our work, you can do so by buying our books or making a direct donation (we are a non-profit/charitable organisation).

office@templelodge.com

TEMPLE LODGE
For the finest books of Science and Spirit